Putting a Name to It

Putting a Name to It
Diagnosis in Contemporary Society

Annemarie Goldstein Jutel
Victoria University of Wellington
Wellington, New Zealand

Foreword by Peter Conrad

The Johns Hopkins University Press
Baltimore

RA
418
.J88
2011

67154012

© 2011 The Johns Hopkins University Press
All rights reserved. Published 2011
Printed in the United States of America on acid-free paper
9   8   7   6   5   4   3   2   1

The Johns Hopkins University Press
2715 North Charles Street
Baltimore, Maryland 21218-4363
www.press.jhu.edu

Library of Congress Cataloging-in-Publication Data

Jutel, Annemarie.
    Putting a name to it : diagnosis in contemporary society / Annemarie
Goldstein Jutel ; foreword by Peter Conrad.
       p. cm.
    Includes bibliographical references and index.
    ISBN-13: 978–1–4214–0067–9 (hardcover : alk. paper)
    ISBN-10: 1–4214–0067–7 (hardcover : alk. paper)
    1. Social medicine. 2. Diagnosis—Social aspects. I. Title.
    RA418.J88 2011
    362.1—dc22   2010042464

A catalog record for this book is available from the British Library.

Special discounts are available for bulk purchases of this book. For more informa-
tion, please contact Special Sales at 410-516-6936 or specialsales@press.jhu.edu.

The Johns Hopkins University Press uses environmentally friendly book
materials, including recycled text paper that is composed of at least 30
percent post-consumer waste, whenever possible. All of our book papers
are acid-free, and our jackets and covers are printed on paper with recycled
content.

To my parents, Samuel Joseph Goldstein, Jr., and Carol Hirschler Goldstein

Contents

Foreword, by Peter Conrad   *ix*
Preface   *xi*

Introduction: What's in a Name?   1
A Place for a Sociology of Diagnosis? 5
An Avenue for Understanding 12

1   Lumping or Splitting: Classification in Medical Diagnosis   15
The Aims of Classification 18
Classification of Diseases 20
Classification Systems 26
Revealing Classificatory Politics in Diagnosis 35

2   Social Framing and Diagnosis: Corpulence and Fetal Death   39
Corpulence 42
Fetal Death 51
Frame and Be Framed 59

3   What's Wrong with Me? Diagnosis and the
Patient-Doctor Relationship   62
Illness and Disease 63
Medical Authority 67
Changing Roles in Diagnosis 68
What Next? 73

4   Beyond Our Ken? Contested Diagnoses and the
Medically Unexplained   76
Medically Unexplained Symptoms 80
Discovery of Disease 87
Whose Diagnosis? 93
Splitting from Diagnosis? 95

5   Driving Diagnosis: Peddlers and Pushers   97
     Engines of Diagnosis 99
     Female Hypoactive Sexual Desire Disorder 102
     Discussion 112

6   "There Is Nothing So Small as to Escape Our Inquiry":
     Technologies of Diagnosis   117
     Technology and Diagnostic Categories 118
     Technology and the Diagnostic Process 122
     Screening 126
     Hope 132

     Conclusion: Directions for the Sociology of Diagnosis   136
     Creation 139
     Application 140
     Allocation 140
     Exploitation 141
     Moving Forward 142

     Notes   147
     References   149
     Index   171

Foreword

Diagnosis constitutes the naming of an ailment or condition based on classifications that are embedded in extant medical knowledge. Diagnosis is a critical feature of medicine, simultaneously identifying what is wrong, providing a roadmap for treatment options, and assessing possible outcomes or prognoses. As the physician Michael Balint noted, diagnosis transforms apparently random symptoms into an organized illness. Although diagnosis is an emblematic medical event, Annemarie Jutel shows in this important book that it is also an event with significant social roots and consequences.

The process and impact of diagnosis has been an object of sociological study for decades, but that study has not necessarily manifestly focused on the development and application of the diagnosis itself. What Jutel does here is bring together numerous strands of sociological work and link them to articulate the social construction, framing, meaning, application, and consequences of medical diagnosis. Some faces of diagnosis will be familiar to social scientists; others are new and fresh.

While reading this book I was reminded how diagnosis, in other frames, has been significant to my own research. For example, the process of medicalization—the development of medical categories for previously nonmedical problems—is an important part of studying the development and consequences of diagnosis. We can often see different groups promoting or resisting diagnostic categories. Diagnoses have histories and can reflect cultural settings. What happened to hysteria, and how did obesity become an illness? Social circumstances may matter as well. Three decades ago, in a study of the experience of epilepsy, the meaning of diagnosis emerged as central to illness experience. We encountered individuals with a new diagnosis of epilepsy. For some it was "Oh no, my life is ruined, who will marry me, who will employ me?" while others responded, "It's only epilepsy, whew, what a relief, I was worried it was a brain tumor." We have the same diagnosis with divergent consequences.

Other sociologists have examined contested illness—that is, lay versus professional contention over the reality of a disease, in cases like chronic fatigue syndrome or fibromyalgia—which are essentially battles over diagnosis. Diagnosis is the gateway to the sick role and whatever benefits can be derived; for some it can provide impetus for biographical change, because not only do individuals have a disease or disorder but their diagnosis may also become part of their identity, legitimizing their life situation. Diagnosis may be key for individuals to obtain medical care and insurance reimbursement for their ailments. And, given that the attribution of diagnosis is a human endeavor, misdiagnosis and medical error remain possibilities with serious consequences.

This book examines the social nature and consequences of diagnosis, whether they be in pharmaceutical promotion, in the technologies used to justify and support diagnoses, or in the medical battles over diagnosis. Jutel has done us all a service by drawing our attention to the sociological centrality of diagnosis and showing us analytical levers for understanding the ways diagnosis shapes medicine, illness, and care. This book is a welcome consolidation and redirection for future sociological studies of diagnosis.

Peter Conrad
Harry Coplan Professor of Social Sciences
Brandeis University

Preface

I don't get sick very often. In fact, as I write these pages, I can't remember the last time I had a cold. But like most mortals, I have been sick before. One particular bout of illness marked me more than others. It was more than 20 years ago, but I remember things well. I had a low-grade fever, enlarged lymph nodes under my arms and in my groin, a strange swelling on my lower leg, and headaches. These symptoms persisted for days, lengthening to weeks, and I couldn't go to work. I was a nurse in a medical oncology unit, and to have a fever made me a risk to my immunocompromised patients.

I went to the HMO to find out what was wrong. "It's nothing," the doctor told me and sent me home to stew. But I didn't get better. A week went by and the fever persisted. It didn't seem right that I (she-who-is-never-ill) would not bounce back more quickly. So I went back to see the doctor. "Could it be the yuppie flu, or something like that?" I ventured, having read about this curious disorder in the paper. "Of course, it couldn't!" she snapped at me. "Didn't I tell you to just wait this out?" I didn't know that much of the medical world refuted the existence of "yuppie flu" or that many doctors were irritated by the lay interest in the disorder. She signed my sick leave form nonetheless, and I slunk away, castigated.

Listless and a bit confused, I decided to leave the city and stay with my mom and dad. My husband drove me and the children to the town where I grew up. I paid an immediate visit to the family practice I had attended since high school, thinking that the doctors there would be kinder and maybe more helpful. The young resident who saw me was immediately as concerned as I was about my illness. I pulled up my pant leg and showed him my lump, making a half-hearted joke about "my tumor." He couldn't hide his surprise as he looked at the raised and angry bump on my shin that had looked for weeks like a permanent almost-bruise. "I think it would be a good idea to try to rule out malignancy," he said, as blunt as you like. On one hand, he shocked me badly.

On the other, he finally spoke to what had been bothering me for more than two weeks. What was the meaning of this illness? Was I going to be OK?

His concern took me on a long journey to find the name for what ailed me. Without a diagnosis, I was rudderless. What did it mean to have all these symptoms, not knowing what they were? Did I have lymphoma, or something worse? Would I see my children grow up? Or was I simply having troubles shaking a viral infection, something just a bit more tenacious than usual? Without a diagnosis, I had no way of understanding my condition, what to expect, even where to turn for support.

X-rays, biopsies, skin tests, and blood work assembled a clearer picture. The lump became *erythema nodosum;* the enlarged lymph nodes, *noncaseating granuloma;* the illness, *sarcoidosis. Sarcoidosis* was a new word for me, not part of my vocabulary. And because this news was delivered in the pre-Internet era, I couldn't quietly hunker down in front of a screen and follow a hundred different trails to information about the condition and its implications. Despite being a health professional, I didn't know how to find out more other than by asking my doctor or talking to my doctor friends. I would have had to venture to the medical library, a foreign land, and rummage about, hoping no one would take me for the imposter I would have felt I was.

The ignorance gave way to fear when my enthusiastic young resident, who had unsettled me previously with his blunt acknowledgment of potential malignancy, just as bluntly told me that people die from sarcoidosis. Either it comes on chronically and progresses, he explained, or it begins acutely but then recedes. Was this acute? I wondered, thinking about the low-grade symptoms I had experienced. Neither the doctor nor I had an answer to that question, although today, with 20 years hindsight, we know it was. The fear, in time, receded, and I carried my diagnosis away with me.

The diagnosis played an important role in the way I understand my life and understood my illness. Prediagnosis, I could neither explain, cure, nor palliate my physical ailments. The pursuit of the diagnosis was a pursuit of organization and explanation, one that required external support. Without medical support, I couldn't sign my own sick forms or justify why I couldn't work.

Once delivered, the diagnosis offered more than simply clarification. It allayed my anxiety (albeit while introducing new ones, at least in the short term) and directed my care. But it also conferred a new identity. In the moment of the diagnosis, I became someone with an autoimmune disorder. Even 20 years later, this label accompanies me to my doctor's appointments, makes the doctor anxious when I cough (lung symptoms are the "bad" ones in sarcoidosis), and explains the blips on the radar: the chronically low white blood-cell count, the occasional photophobia.

This journey, this experience of illness, banal in its configuration, punctuates the importance that diagnosis plays in understanding health and illness. Labeling disease makes an important contribution to social structure and to individual experiences. In the case of my interactions, it defined my role and that of my doctors. The diagnosis legitimized my illness, giving me access to laboratory tests and medicine. The doctor's ability to diagnose gave him power: authorized the allocation of resources, of sick leave, and of the label. The pursuit of the diagnosis structured my interaction with the medical corps. It instigated the consultation and stayed at the fore as we (doctor and patient) worked together to arrive at a label that made sense within our respective clinical and lived experiences.

The social impact of having a particular diagnosis is considerable. Beyond its organizational role and the access it provides to resources, diagnosis can stigmatize as well as legitimize, with psychiatry often guarding the boundaries between deviance and disease. Unexplained physical distress is often expressed as a psychiatric diagnosis. With few exceptions, only the medical profession has the power to diagnose disease; this medical custodianship of diagnosis reinforces medical authority. It defines which specialty should assume responsibility for which disorders and sets the groundwork for social communication.

Diagnoses themselves emerge from social contexts. Before a condition can become a disease, it must be perceived to be undesirable and it must be visible. That dementia should not be present in middle-aged people was an important prerequisite for being able to name Alzheimer disease, as was the development of diagnostic technology that enabled researchers to distinguish the neurological abnormalities of that disease from other brain disorders. Technology frames new diagnoses and effaces others, while research agendas, commercial interests, and lay activism also help shape which diseases are recognized and which treatments are publicized and promoted.

The studies that have been made of diagnosis have been more predictably studies of diagnoses—one disease at a time. The sociology of diagnosis has been concealed within a range of different disciplines (history and philosophy of medicine, medical sociology, anthropology, and so on) not clearly revealed for concerted scrutiny. In this book, I try to palliate this situation, providing an opportunity to study myriad topics from the diagnostic perspective: patient-doctor interaction, medicalization, illness experiences, health social movements, disease recognition, and others. This analysis reveals the layers of negotiation, compromise, and interests that frame diseases and their consequences.

Mildred Blaxter wrote one of the earliest sociological analyses of diagnosis as a cultural artifact in her 1978 article about alcoholism. She described the fact that diagnosis is both the preexisting set of categories agreed on by the medical profession to designate a specific condition it considers pathological and the process, or deliberate judgment, by which such a label is applied (Blaxter 1978). At the same time, the process and the category are intertwined, making it difficult to speak of one without considering the other. While it might be convenient to divide this book into two parts, one focusing on diagnosing, and the other on diagnostic categories, I have opted instead to weave the two together, recognizing that other analytic approaches are possible. In any case, the scholar of diagnosis should keep in mind (where I might fail to explicitly acknowledge it) that no disease exists in isolation from the way in which it is conferred to those who have the disease.

In the following pages, my path starts from an introduction that presents a broad picture of the social nature of medical diagnosis. I expose in general terms how diagnosis is framed by society and culture and how, in turn, it frames the experience of illness.

In chapter 1, I outline the role of classification in understanding the social context and implications of diagnosis. The classifications into which doctors and lay people slot their explanations of illness determine much about the disease yet reveal little about the production of the classification itself: the principles involved, the voices present, and interests satisfied as well as those silenced and disappointed.

Chapter 1 explores the goals of classification and its embodiment in medical diagnosis. I provide a brief overview of the aims and principles of classification and their relevance to medicine. I demonstrate how classifications operate as social framing devices that enable and disable communication, assert and refute authority, and are important items for sociological study.

In chapter 2 I undertake an in-depth look at two specific diagnoses. I explore the cultural context in which these diagnoses come to validate what decision makers are able to consider. We see how a diagnosis is cast as a reality simply waiting to be labeled. This speaks to Hacking's (2001) comments on the intense interest in the classification of people. The focus is on "a picture of an object to be searched out, the right classification, the classification that is true to nature, a fixed target if only we can get there" (p. 11). I use two tangible physical conditions as a basis for this chapter (overweight and fetal death) to focus on how conditions that are clinically measurable are nonetheless not spared from social content, contests, and consequences.

Overweight, I argue, is a new condition that can be framed as a diagnosis only in a social context in which scales are available to determine body weight (in distinction to qualitative "fatness") and in which there is a prevailing confidence in the ability of statistical assessment of weight to assess individual health. I show how weight has become assimilated as a proxy measure of well-being in Western society, a practice that was initially strongly resisted and remains dubious.

Through my review of the terms *abortion, miscarriage,* and *stillbirth,* I underline the implications embodied in the diagnostic terms used to designate fetal death and describe how they establish conflicting subject positions for mother and fetus. I also examine the statutory regulations that affirm the problematic terms, drawing on specific examples from New Zealand, while recognizing similarities across Western cultures.

Chapter 3 explores the links between the lay-professional relationship and diagnosis. The diagnosis provides a rationale for the consultation, confirms the authority and prestige of the medical profession, delegates the responsibility for labeling an illness, and in our contemporary era provides access to a range of resources. The diagnosis is generally a prerequisite for treatment, an imperative for reimbursement, an authorization to deviate from expected behaviors—in sum, a legitimating force. This chapter explores the role of diagnosis in the doctor-patient relationship, describing the differences evidenced in, and created by, the illness-disease dichotomy and the tensions and goals of the encounter.

The tensions present in the doctor-patient relationship are most pronounced in the case of contested diagnoses and medically unexplained symptoms. Chapter 4 describes how the absence of diagnosis changes the nature of the patient-doctor relationship. It simultaneously tests the credibility of the doctor and the patient—the former for his or her inability to label the patient's complaint and the latter for the ignominy of being perceived to have a factitious symptom. This chapter discusses patient-doctor tension in the diagnostic process, notably when there is misalignment between the medical and lay assessment of illness. This tension is often present when a medical explanation cannot be found for what an individual clearly believes to be physical illness. I explore how medicine manages that which it cannot explain and discuss why this is frequently unacceptable to lay people who believe they are ill. I will look at how diseases come to be recognized by medicine and the role that lay people play (or are prevented from playing) as ailments gain official recognition of their status as legitimate diseases.

Chapter 5 borrows Peter Conrad's notion of "engines" to describe forces outside of medicine that promote and give life to particular diagnostic categories. I use as a heuristic the relatively obscure diagnosis of female hypoactive sexual desire disorder, which is currently surfacing in medical and marketing literature as a frequent disorder worthy of concern. I describe how this diagnosis embodies long-standing fascination with female libido, a contemporary focus on female hypersexuality, and commercial interest of the pharmaceutical industry and its medical allies to reify low sexual urge as a pathological disorder. To understand the way diagnoses are promoted by nonmedical sources requires reflection not only on the pharmaceutical industry but other industries, as well as the context in which diagnosis currently takes place.

In Chapter 6, I explore the technologies of diagnosis. Technology underpins many diagnoses. From genetic screening to sophisticated visual imaging, a range of tools enable medicine to identify previously silent risk factors and other latent processes. Technology enables "surrogate markers" (such as laboratory results) to act as a proxy for clinical events. It also opens the way for the discussion of genetic probability, with its significant bioethical consequences. This chapter discusses the importance of technology in the sociology of diagnosis and technology's contribution to both understanding and obfuscating the clinical.

The conclusion draws together the many threads that are introduced and developed in the foregoing chapters. Its purpose is to synthesize these in order to develop a model for understanding and studying diagnosis in its social complexity. I propose directions for the field to consider diagnosis as an object of sociological study, while inviting further discussion and debate.

Some of the material in this book has been present in other forms in my earlier publications: "Does Size Really Matter?" (2001), "Weighing Health" (2005), "The Emergence of Overweight as a Disease Entity" (2006a), "What's in a Name?" (2006b), "Medicine's Flight from Interpretation" (2007), "Doctor's Orders" (2008), "Framing Disease" (2010a), and "Medically Unexplained Symptoms and the Disease Label" (2010b).

I could not have written this book without assistance, and I would like to thank the many people who have contributed to my effort. My colleagues in Dunedin, Wellington, and farther afield read many drafts and listened patiently to my raging torrent of consciousness: Deborah Davis, Jenny Aimers, Kevin Dew, and David Menkes. Many new e-friends and colleagues were willing to meet in cyberspace (and occasionally in person) and have generously given their feedback and support: Phil Brown, Allan Horwitz, Peter Conrad, Joel Lexchin, and particularly Sarah Nettleton. I am grateful to my incredible research assistant, John Gardner, and my just-as-incredible literary advisor, Sue Wootton, and to Douglas Booth, my mentor, advisor, and supervisor since undergraduate days. My punctilious and creative sister, Ellen Goldstein; my dear friend Alison Bradshaw; my ever-patient light and life partner, Thierry Jutel; my beautiful children, Olivier Jutel and Mélanie Piri, and their families, who have provided me with joy (and even theoretical advice) along the way, deserve special thanks. I would also like to remember my friend Ruth Schick, who read my work in the months before her death. She was generous in her enthusiasm.

Thanks go as well to those anonymous reviewers who have gotten their teeth into my work over the years to help shape my ideas more clearly and make their impact more salient. You know who you are.

Putting a Name to It

Introduction

What's in a Name?

"Has anyone mentioned Huntington's disease to you?" . . .

Baxter is looking at the ground. Perowne takes his silence as confirmation.

"Do you want to tell me who your doctor is?"

"Why would I do that?"

"We could get you referred to a colleague of mine. He's good. He could make things easier for you."

At this, Baxter turns and angles his head in his attempt to settle the taller man's image on his fovea, that small depression on the retina where vision is most acute. There's nothing anyone can do about a damaged saccadic system. And, generally, there's nothing on offer at all for this condition, beyond managing the descent. But Henry sees now in Baxter's agitated features a sudden avidity, a hunger for information, or hope. Or simply a need to talk.

"What sort of thing?"

"Exercises. Certain drugs."

"Exercise . . ." He snorts on the word. He is right to pick up on the futility, the feebleness of the idea. Perowne presses on.

"What has your doctor told you?"   IAN MCEWAN (2004)

The power of the diagnosis is remarkable. Receiving a diagnosis is like being handed a road map in the middle of a forest. It shows the way—but not necessarily the way out. It indicates what the path ahead is going to look like, where it will lead, the difficulty of the climb, and various potential turnoffs along the way. Perhaps it identifies the destination, but not necessarily. With a diagnosis, things don't necessarily get better, but they become clearer. The unexplained becomes explained, and management is defined. Assumptions are made about the future.

The diagnostic moment is simultaneously transformative and contingent.

Its transformative power is captured in the extract at the beginning of this chapter. In McEwan's story, Perowne, a neurosurgeon, makes a sidewalk diagnosis of Huntingon disease in a thug who has started beating him up. His involuntary, uncoordinated, and jerky movements are a dead giveaway. When Perowne names the disorder, his attacker is completely disarmed; the fact of his diagnosis (albeit one he already knew) refocuses the present.

Suzanne Fleischmann (1999), in her poignant linguistic discussion of her own (ultimately fatal) disease, explains that "the verbal act of presenting a patient with a diagnosis is never a simple act of conveying value-neutral biomedical information. It is an act fraught with symbolism. If a person is told 'you have cancer' (or any life-threatening disease) *these words* irrevocably alter that person's consciousness, view of the future, relationships with family and friends, and so on. Moreover, the utterance marks a boundary. It serves to divide a life into 'before' and 'after,' and this division is henceforth superimposed onto every rewrite of the individual's life story" (p. 10).

Even in less dramatic circumstances, diagnosis frames reality in significant ways. Few readers of these pages would not have one day thought, "What would I do if I found I had X?" imagining how life would look if, out of the blue, a serious diagnosis interrupted the quotidian. "Would I even want to know?"

I remember the great ethical debates around *la verité au malade* (telling the truth to patients) when I was a young nursing student in 1980s France. Did health professionals have the right to throw people's lives into disarray by sharing devastating diagnoses with them? Sometimes it was better not to, we were told. I worked at the Clinique Catherine de Sienne—an oncology clinic—where nursing staff were not allowed to pronounce the word *cancer* within earshot of patients. Its effect would be too emotionally devastating. We should leave such diagnoses in medical hands, out of respect for their transformative power.[1] In contrast, when I nursed in medical oncology in the United States for several years, the truth was distributed liberally in its naked, harsh form. In a different culture, rights associated with diagnosis took a different form. With self-determination at the heart of the American dream, knowledge of one's ailment provides the object against which to react, the starting point for self-realization.

The contingency of diagnosis, on the other hand, is generally not as obvious as its transformative power. Diagnoses are presented as facts of nature, yet they hide a deeply grounded, socially negotiated genesis. As real and ob-

servable (and explanatory) as cellular material might be on a glass slide, choosing to look at it (and being able to do so) are contingent on two things: human-
made technology and the assumption that particular symptoms are physical
in nature. We don't, for example, look for "generosity traits" in blood tests,
although nineteenth-century phrenologists and physiognomists sought to confirm their presence in the biophysical.

Diagnosis is always a social creation. That doesn't mean that the diseases it
labels aren't "real," but it does mean that before a diagnosis can exist, it has to
be visible, problematic, and perceived to be related to the field of medicine. All
of these factors are linked to social mores. Dyslexia, as one example, may be
a disorder in the Western world but would not be problematic in a nonliterate
society. What a particular group perceives to be problematic or unacceptable,
needing remedy, is socially contingent.

Diagnosis provides a cultural expression of what a given society is prepared
to accept as normal and what it feels should be treated. We might chuckle to
think that witchcraft (Gevitz 2000) and the tendency of slaves to run away
(drapetomania) (Cartwright 1981) were once seen as diseases, as if we now
had a superior understanding of the true nature of medicine. Many readers
will probably remember when homosexuality was a "disease." While it had, in
one epoch, been seen as perfectly normal and in another as evidence of moral
depravity, its status as a medical concern was solidified by its inscription in
the *Diagnostic and Statistical Manual of Mental Disorders* as a mental disease
(Mendelson 2003).

While witchcraft, drapetomania, and homosexuality bear no relation to
medicine's twenty-first-century sensitivity, the knowing chuckle is misplaced.
It's not the technological advancement of medicine that stops us labeling what
we don't like or understand as disease. It's that we can't easily step out of
our current vantage point to see the cultural content that historical distance
provides.

Might there be similar contemporary examples that will look as droll and
as value laden to those who will read our books and diagnostic manuals one
hundred years hence? Excited delirium would undoubtedly raise a few eyebrows, as would female hypoactive sexual desire disorder. Excited delirium is
a diagnosis that is pronounced most frequently in a coroner's court, when labeling the cause of death of an agitated inmate or patient held under restraint.
This syndrome of death in custody ascribes a pathological origin to an always-
controversial result. Medical scapegoat? Genetic fault? Excited delirium de-

serves careful scrutiny, given the potential it carries for projecting the guilt of overzealous constraint onto pathophysiology (Paquette 2003).

Female hypoactive sexual desire disorder, which I explore in greater depth in chapter 6, might be another source of raised eyebrows for our hypothetical future readers. This diagnosis is applied to women whose lack of sexual desire causes them distress (Clayton et al. 2009). That it exists as a disease category is contingent on unproven beliefs about what constitutes "normal" sexuality. Ah, the elusive "normal"! In other eras, heightened female libido was thought to be an ailment, rather than a normative urge, because "normal" referred to a low sexual drive. Psychiatrists used the term *psychopathic* to describe women who engaged in sexual activity beyond the bounds of what genteel society felt was moral (Lunbeck 1987).

Diagnoses with social content are not just psychiatric, contested, or controversial. Even mundane and observable conditions such as overweight, infertility, and Lyme disease are dependent for their existence on social judgments and beliefs. I discuss each of these in greater depth in subsequent chapters, exposing the surprising lack of evidence about the risks of overweight, the nonmedical alternatives for considering unwanted childlessness, and the convergence of social factors that enabled Lyme disease to be recognized as a disease.

Diagnoses are classification tools. They segment and organize the vast continuum of human conditions. Diagnosis validates what counts as disease and what doesn't, prioritizing some conditions over others and always exerting an important material force (Bowker and Star 1999) as it guides medical care. The diagnosis is interpretive and organizational (Balint 1964). When people visit the doctor to find out "what's wrong," they bring a picture of disarray to the consultation: a collection of symptoms and problems they presume to be medical in nature. The diagnosis provides structure—sorting out the real from the imagined, the valid from the feigned, the significant from the insignificant, the physical from the psychological. Once the diagnosis is made, the concordant treatment can be planned, the prognosis reflected on, and resources allocated. Resources include access to such varied items as medications, physiotherapy sessions, sick leave, specialist referrals, and prostheses. The diagnosis is both rudder and anchor: its pursuit guides the individual to the doctor's consulting rooms, while its assignment positions identity and behavior.

Being diagnosed gives permission to be ill. This is what Parsons (1951) referred to as "a claim for exemption." Prior to the recognition of disease, the individual is not "allowed" to fail in his or her social expectations: getting out of bed and getting dressed, going to work or school, doing housework or looking after the children. The suffering person is excused from these responsibilities once diagnosed and is no longer *blamed* for failing to achieve normative expectations. Instead, he or she is *treated* (Freidson 1970). The diagnosis enables the individual to socially reintegrate, albeit with allowance made for illness and a sanctioned explanation of what makes him or her different from everyone else.

Because of its power to confirm status and allocate resources, the diagnosis is also an important site of contest and compromise. It is a relational process, with each party (lay and medical) confronting illness with different explanations, understandings, values, and beliefs. The misfit between patient and medical explanatory models may result, individually, in unsatisfactory therapeutic values and goals (Kleinman, Eisenberg, and Good 1978). Or, collectively, it may generate politicization of illness, with social movements and disease advocacy groups battling for recognition, funding, and other forms of support (P. Brown and Zavestoski 2004).

A Place for a Sociology of Diagnosis?

Despite the influential role of diagnosis in medicine and in lay-professional relations, it does not have its own sociology, literature, or disciplinary focus. Phil Brown (1990) called for a sociology of diagnosis many years ago, arguing that diagnosis was only loosely studied by sociologists, notwithstanding the fact that so doing would provide an important insight into how we comprehend disease, health, illness, and the forces that shape our knowledge and practices. The studies that have been made of diagnosis have been more predictably studies of diagnoses—one label in isolation from another, serving as a heuristic or example of medicalization, disease theory, or history of disease. It's not that diagnosis has been excluded from medical sociology. It's simply that it has been concealed inside these and other areas of focus and hasn't been clearly isolated to be explored on its own. Extirpating diagnosis and revealing it for specific discussion provides an opportunity to study an array of topics from a different perspective: for example, patient-doctor interaction, medicalization, illness experiences, health social movements, disease recognition, and more.

In the chapters of this book I lay bare some of the important cornerstones of the sociology of diagnosis. Each section analyzes, from a different perspective, the specific role of diagnosis in medical sociology. The book cannot define the field, but it will start the ball rolling, drawing together a number of threads of medical sociology that potentially contribute to the development of this important subdiscipline.

Diagnosis and Medical Identity

Thomas Willis is the first person known to have used the term *diagnosis*, which he defined as "Dilucidation, or Knowledg" in a work published in 1681. He must have used the term previously, as this definition occurs in his posthumous "remaining" works. He had died in 1675. By 1701, the Reverend George William Lemon referred to "diagnostics" [qui est dignoscendi, peritus: subtle discerner]: "A knowledge or judgment of the apparent signs of a distemper, or a skill by which the present condition of a distemper is perceived, and this is three-fold, *viz.* 1. A right judgment of the part affected. 2. Of the disease itself. 3. Of its case."

This does not mean that before these writings medical practitioners did not seek to differentiate one ailment from another. Around the time that Willis wrote his definition, changes were afoot in the way medicine considered disease. At the start of the eighteenth century, a classification movement was in full swing, with naturalists from Europe sailing the world, exploring, collecting, and categorizing the living world. The idea was that taxonomy would provide a mechanism for understanding the world and for understanding and celebrating God's presence on Earth. As one mother wrote in a little textbook for her children, "We have reviewed all the classes of beings from insects to man, and we have recognized the hand of God everywhere. We have seen everywhere order and harmony which force our admiration. It would be impossible for us in the face of all these marvels of nature, not to praise He who created all" (Anon. 1840, p. 72).

Medicine followed the natural sciences and engaged in the great classificatory project that would underpin diagnosis. I discuss this further in chapter 2. Classification would identify the features that distinguished one disease from another and the tools by which an individual doctor might assign a particular disease label. It would also offer a means by which the profession could consolidate itself. Classification provided—among other things—the language for discussing matters of collective concern and for passing along medical knowledge.

Just as it provided a focus for medicine to consolidate itself, diagnosis also provided a mechanism for discerning the lay from the professional. Being able to diagnose is at the base of the social authority afforded the doctor. It sets the doctor apart from the lay person and from other professionals, confirming the doctor's greater knowledge and status (Freidson 1970). Diagnosis also structures relationships within the profession, defining who should assume responsibility for particular disorders (Rosenberg 2002): this complaint to the general practitioner, that one to the immunologist, the hematologist, or the rheumatologist. Particular branches of medicine have used diagnosis to confirm their credibility. Much has been written of the extent to which the *Diagnostic and Statistical Manual of Mental Disorders*, psychiatry's bible, became a tool by which the discipline was able to assert its authority at a time when many other professions were encroaching on psychiatry's domain. I discuss this in greater depth in the pages to come.

Diagnoses and their classificatory systems are an important collective arrangement that defines and enables the promotion of professional medicine. The authority of medicine, according to de Swaan (1989), resides in such professional accords about scientific medicine.

At an individual level, the ability to assign a diagnosis also confers power to medicine and its agent, the doctor, as allocator of resources (de Swaan 1989). The diagnosis legitimizes sickness. As discussed previously, when a doctor deems a patient's condition to be medical, the latter receives previously unauthorized privileges, such as permission to be absent from work, priority parking, reimbursement for treatment, or access to services. The doctor certifies the medical nature of the complaint, and "medical advice" informs administrative and policy decisions.

Freidson's (1970) work on professional dominance focuses on the important role of diagnosis in reinforcing medical authority. It is, he postulates, "the . . . foundation upon which the strength of a profession rests . . . which establishes and supports the profession's claim to honor, income and power. Where illness is the ubiquitous label for deviance in an age, the profession that is custodian of the label is ascendent" (p. 244). He continues: diagnosis is the mission of the doctor, whose task is "to authoritatively label as illness what a complainant suspects to be illness, and also to label as illness what was not previously labeled at all, or what was labelled in some other fashion, under some other institution's jurisdiction" (p. 261).

Authority in medicine comes from its ability to define and delimit behaviors, persons, and conditions, write Peter Conrad and Joseph Schneider (1980). But it also derives from the organization and structure of the medical profession. Medicine has an officially approved monopoly over the right to define health and to treat illness, which results in its high public esteem (Freidson 1970). Doctors have historically held, and still hold today, a prominent role in both the health and general social hierarchy, with particular credibility given to their ways of knowing about the body.

That being said, medical and lay roles are dynamic and are currently in flux. Access to information once restricted to medical professionals places the lay person in a different position relative to medicine's authority. The expert patient can now discuss, challenge, and contest the medical dominance. In some instances, it must be said, medicine willingly (and perhaps surprisingly) relinquishes ownership of the diagnosis to the patient. For example, a sub-classification of migraine in the *International Statistical Classification of Diseases and Related Health Problems* is "intractable migraine, *so-stated*" (emphasis added). For this diagnosis to exist, the patient must speak (Bowker and Star 1999). And during the recent H1N1 pandemic, diagnostic authority was offered to lay people in the interest of infection control. Public health messages asked people to stay at home if they had the flu, thus promoting self-diagnosis of the disease.

The authority to diagnose some medical conditions has also been expanded to include other professional categories. In New Zealand, for example, a chiropractor or physiotherapist may diagnose certain conditions and grant access to Accident Compensation Corporation benefits and services.

This is not to say that medicine no longer has authority. The biomedical expertise of those trained to practice medicine still carries much weight (Lupton 1997b). The practice of medicine, as well as its authority, is socially contingent and is framed by broader sociotechnological change. Nettleton (2004) discusses this change. She speaks of the informatization of medicine, in which the body is seen as a system of information networks: the art of medicine gives way to evidence-based practice, the physical body defers to the CT scan, information once restricted to medicine is now available to the lay Web surfer, and the doctor-patient relationship becomes a meeting of experts. Medicine's jurisdiction is shifting, incorporating new agents and social forces into its contemporary context. The theory of medicalization offers an explanatory framework to understand the changing yet persistent face of medical authority.

Medicalization is the process by which aspects of human existence are assigned to the realm of medicine, to be defined and managed by medicine's authority. Zola (1972) contended that diagnosis plays an important role in medicalization: "If anything can be shown in some way to effect the workings of the body, and to a lesser extent the mind, then it can be labeled an 'illness' itself or jurisdictionally 'a medical problem'" (p. 495), he wrote. He marveled at the increasing rate of clinical entities and disorders reported in surveys and studies. This close relationship between medicalization and diagnosis may be the fundamental explanation of why a sociology of diagnosis has not had its own delineation: it has been enveloped in the folds of medicalization.

This broader literature of medicalization informs the sociology of diagnosis by the way in which it establishes the authoritative and pervasive position of medicine in Western society. Conrad's later definition points to the role of diagnosis in medicalization, indicating the place of illness and disorders in the assertion of medicine's professional territory. But medicalization encompasses more than just diagnosis. For example, infant feeding and child rearing have been—and continue to be—medicalized as part of scientific motherhood (Apple 1995). The privileging of medical authority over other forms of knowledge (even when there is no diagnosis or pathological condition) is notably present in parenting, where the mother or father might seek medical advice for matters of infant health, using medical endorsement for child nutrition and educational products, and reading doctor-authored columns or books on childrearing. In contrast, sadness, say, or sexual problems, both arguably nonmedical in nature, are variably transformed by the diagnostic labels "depression" and "erectile dysfunction," triggering an array of medicalized reactions. In these cases, the diagnosis is a specific step into, and an enabling factor of, medicalization.

Understanding medicalization requires us to look at the work of earlier social scientists who were concerned with medicine's authority in contemporary society and its role in legitimizing social concerns (Zola 1983). Before the emergence of the concept of medicalization, Parsons (1951, 1979) and Freidson (1970) wrote about the roles of the various components of the social system. Freidson focused particularly on the professional role of the physician with regard to illness, while Parsons explored health and illness in terms of how they affected participation in a social system. "Health and illness," he wrote, "are not only 'conditions' or 'states' of the human individual . . . they are also states evaluated and institutionally recognized in the culture and social structure of societies" (1979, p. 126).

Zola acknowledged that one of the means by which medicalization functions is by affixing diagnostic labels to socially deviant behavior. Conrad and Schneider (P. Conrad 1975, 1979, 1992; P. Conrad and Schneider, 1980) explore this in greater depth, most notably in their coauthored book *Deviance and Medicalization: From Badness to Sickness* (1980). They note the role of medicine in reform—medical crusaders attempting to influence public morality and behavior—as well as the respect for medical advances. These authors propose a five-stage model by which a deviant behavior is medicalized through diagnoses: defining the behavior as deviant; discovering the behavior from within the medical community; making claims; challenging the existing designation to bring the behavior to medical turf; and institutionalizing the behavior via diagnosis.

A number of scholars focus on the myriad of social conditions receiving medical attention and diagnostic labels. John Rosecrance (1985) extends Conrad and Schneider's model to his work on compulsive gambling. Scholars have explored hyperactivity (P. Conrad 1975), alcoholism (Blaxter 1978), menstruation (Smith-Rosenberg and Rosenberg 1973; Vertinsky 1994), pregnancy (Barker 1998), sexuality (Tiefer 1996), obesity (Jutel 2008), andropause (P. Conrad 2007), adult ADHD (P. Conrad 1979), and even compulsive buying (Lee and Mysyk 2004). These are all examples of the transfer of life events and ways of being to the auspices of medical care.

The expansion of diagnostic categories is not without risk and can have severe iatrogenic results. The treatment that accompanies a diagnosis may expose an individual to undesirable or unintended secondary effects. As one example, the medicalization of shyness, which results in the diagnoses of social phobia, social anxiety disorder, and avoidant personality disorder, encourages patients to request, and doctors to recommend, the use of pharmaceutical remedies, some of which have resulted in reports of devastating side effects (S. Scott 2006). As I note in chapter 5, this focus on diagnosis provides a fertile ground for the commercial exploitation of patients and doctors alike.

Diagnosis and Lay Identity

While diagnosis might arrange and consolidate the identity of the profes-sional, it is more likely to *re*arrange individual identity, threatening previous self-definition as the individual now "inhabits" an illness (Klinkenborg 1994, p. 79). For the person who has a serious or chronic disease, "illness becomes a trope for new attitudes toward the self; it also influences perceptions of that self by others, including, notably, employers and insurers" (Fleischman 1999, p. 13).

An individual narrative of disease is not, however, independent of the *re-gime* associated with a diagnosis, proposes Klawiter (2004). A disease regime is the cultural, spatial, and historical practices associated with a diagnosis, and it goes beyond the circumstances of the individual and the physiologi-cal nature of the illness. Klawiter demonstrates how the narrative of one in-dividual altered over time, as a result of different conditions in which she experienced two separate diagnoses of breast cancer. The agendas, identities, social relations, policies, and emotional vocabularies embodied in different "regimes of practice" around breast cancer transformed public discourses and other forms of cultural production and in turn transformed the narrative of the individual.

Diagnosis may also create collective identities, removing the individual from the isolation of his or her suffering and providing the person with new potential networks of support. In turn, this collective identity has political po-tential to shape, and in some cases challenge, professional authority, political imperatives, and social identity (P. Brown and Zavestoski 2004). Phil Brown (1995) has written about how diagnosis offers a tool for political engagement. Diagnoses such as post-traumatic stress disorder, black lung, and environmen-tal disease offer a social view for victims of abuse or toxic exposure, opening the door to care and to compensation.

Collective identity may be virtual. A growing number of Internet commu-nities are focused on diagnoses. Web pages play a part in the social health movement: gathering individuals around both existing and emerging diseases. Dumit (2006) explains that Internet communities offer a means of survival for those who have medically unexplained symptoms. They provide an alter-native support structure when the absence of diagnosis impugns the medical legitimacy of the individual's complaint.

In any case, the question of identity—which diagnosis (or its absence) helps to consolidate—is important in the social context of health, illness, and disease. It is at the base of lay health movements, it infiltrates doctor-patient relationships, and it is part of how individuals make sense of their illness and its impact on their day-to-day experiences.

An Avenue for Understanding

Medicine is temporally situated, and it makes its diagnoses on the basis of the technology and values available at a given time. As an unidentified writer wrote in the *British Medical Journal* in 1886, "The imperfection of our medical vocabulary is not a matter for surprise. It is the measure and gauge of the imperfection of our medical knowledge, and only perfect knowledge admits of a perfect nomenclature" (Anon. 1886, p. 1116).

Ivan Illich wrote that "disease always intensifies stress, defines incapacity, imposes inactivity, and focuses apprehension on nonrecovery, on uncertainty, and on one's dependence upon future medical findings." He continued: "Once a society organizes for a preventative disease-hunt, it gives epidemic proportions to diagnosis. This ultimate triumph of therapeutic culture turns the independence of the average healthy person into an intolerable form of deviance" (1976, p. 104).

Goode wrote in a similar tone, pointing out that "by devising a linguistic category with specific connotations, one is designing the armaments for a battle; by having it accepted and used, one has scored a major victory" (1969, p. 89). The power of the diagnosis is its classificatory functions: the diagnosis does the work of "making it appear that science describes nature (and nature alone) and that politics is about social power (and social power alone)" (Bowker and Star 1999, p. 46). However, the work of the diagnosis is often invisible, "erased by [its] naturalization into the routines of life," concealing conflict and multiplicity beneath layers of obscure representation (Bowker and Star 1999, p. 47).

Most readers of this book have, at some point, gone to see the doctor to "find out what's wrong." Some go with trepidation, wondering if they're wasting the doctor's time ("It's probably nothing"), while others leave with even more unease than when they went in ("If nothing's wrong with me, why do I feel this way?"). Yet a third group leaves a consultation with a clear sense of what is remiss, instructions about treatment, and, with some luck, an anticipation of when and how the ailment will resolve. Diagnosis structures the reality of individuals, as it clarifies and sometimes explains what they experience. Interactions in the doctor's rooms are strongly framed by what it means both to be a patient and to be a doctor. Subservience to medical authority is both reassuring and problematic. Good patients show signs of "compliance" with and "adherence" to doctor's orders. Informed self-advocates work hard with, and sometimes against, the doctor, probing and questioning why their complaint is or isn't considered medical and protesting if a psychogenic cause is proposed: less physical, less real.

In today's world, where information abounds, the diagnostic relationship between patient and doctor has changed. Patients may, at odds with Balint's description, propose a diagnosis rather than an ailment when they consult. Or they may circumvent the doctor altogether. They calculate their body mass index, take depression self-tests, or use medical terminology to describe their idiosyncrasies and those of their friends. "Are you sure you don't have ADD?" they might quiz, even able to use a readily recognizable acronym for attention deficit disorder. Lay people are changing the shape of what diagnosis means in practice.

The "modern" patient is the ideal: an informed "consumer" who can sit on an equal platform with the doctor as a result of now-open access to information previously restricted to doctors. The idealized clinical encounter is a cooperative interaction that brings patient and doctor together in a kind of handshake agreement about what ails the former and what the latter can do in response. It is not always so simple, particularly as the encounter is about far more, as Hunter (1991) points out, than a simple classification of our malady; focusing on the diagnosis draws attention away from the care of the person who is ill. Furthermore, the profession's acknowledgments of its limitations, as well as of myriad social influences on its classificatory practices, needs attention from within.

Exploring the social forces that influence the clinical process of diagnosis provides a greater understanding of both the fluidity and the fallibility of the diagnosis. Diagnoses do not exist ontologically. They are concepts that bind the biological, the technological, the social, the political, and the lived. Thomas Laqueur wrote that "believing is seeing." Despite the advent of autopsy and a presumed clear vision of the ways in which structures were connected, Renaissance anatomists still depicted the vagina as an inside-out penis and menstrual flow as transformed into breast milk during lactation (Laqueur 1990). Similarly, diagnosis captures what the medical institution currently believes to be "the way things are." Suffice to say, the world of facts is not detachable from an a priori conceptual framework.

Sociology of diagnosis is an important avenue for understanding not only lay experience of illness and lay-professional discord, as I discuss above, but also patient compliance, disease control, public health, health education, and many other aspects of health and illness. Kleinman and colleagues' claims of thirty years ago hold strong today: understanding social science is necessary to deal competently with essential nonbiomedical aspects of clinical practice. They maintain that medicine is both a biological and a social science (Kleinman, Eisenberg, and Good 1978). Focusing on both social and biological aspects assists clinicians to treat patients as well as diseases, a sometimes neglected feature of contemporary medical practice (see Leder 1990; A. Goldstein 2007). Understanding the social frames within which diagnoses are generated and grasping the impact of the label is clinically powerful. As Aronowitz (2001) cautions, there is an "essential continuity between persons who have symptoms that have been given a name and disease-like status and persons whose suffering remains unnamed and unrecognized" (p. 808).

Sociology of diagnosis has a salient role to play in understanding health, illness, and disease: unpacking and identifying the play of interests that enter into discussions of what priorities should be set and what goals attained. Diagnosis defines the field of medicine and its professional reach, serves as the nexus in which the clinical encounter takes place, arbitrates normality and difference, organizes a patient's illness, and determines how resources are allocated. In this introduction I have, with a broad brush, covered a range of considerations that contribute to a sociology of diagnosis: the place of naming in medicine and the tensions naming can engender. But there is more work to be done. A rich collection of structures, agents, and actions enter into the diagnostic arena and deserve consideration. Identifying, analyzing, and understanding these and their connections will ultimately contribute to a better understanding of medicine's role and how it achieves it, as well as the relationship of medicine to culture and society.

Lumping or Splitting

Classification in Medical Diagnosis

> We are not to suppose that there are only a certain number of divisions in
> any subject, and that unless we follow these, we shall divide it wrongly and
> unsuccessfully: on the contrary every subject is as it were all joints, it will
> divide wherever we choose to strike it, and therefore according to our par-
> ticular object at different times we shall see fit to divide it very differently.
>
> THOMAS ARNOLD (1839)

D iagnosis is one of medicine's most powerful classification tools. Understanding classification must be part of the quest to understand the social
context and implications of diagnosis more clearly. Classification provides a
foundation for the recognition and study of illness: deciding how the vast
expanse of nature can be partitioned into meaningful chunks, stabilizing and
structuring what is otherwise disordered. The classifications into which doctors and lay people slot their explanations of illness determine much about
disease. Yet little is revealed about how these classifications are produced, the
principles involved, the voices present and interests satisfied, or those silenced
and disappointed.

Effective classification recognizes difference as well as similarity. By classifying, we are putting items together that have more in common with one
another than they do with things we have decided belong in another category
(Zerubavel 1996). There needs to be a reasonable rationale for placing similar
objects together, ensuring that there is enough resemblance among members
of the category for them to be associated, while not obfuscating difference.
This is the principle of Ockham's razor: "entities are not to be multiplied be-

yond necessity" (*entia non sunt multiplicanda praeter necessitatem entia non sunt multiplicanda praeter necessitatem*) (Ockham, William of 1997). Okham's principle highlights simplicity: don't get too complex when a few general categories will do.

But the rationale for classifying is always fluid, as Arnold adumbrates in the epigraph to this chapter. Subjects are "all joints," he says, pointing out that the "various branches of human knowledge are capable of the most different arrangements according to the light in which we wish to regard them" (pp. 5–6).

Arnold used "the vegetable creation" to describe the opportunistic nature of classification. If we are to classify vegetables in relation to people, he explained, we might put wheat, potatoes, and figs in the same conceptual basket. These are all products of the vegetable kingdom that are *edible* for humans. On the other hand, if we are concerned with their botanical taxonomy, the classification changes: grasses, tubers, and trees become the organizing principles of these clusters. We'll put wheat and flax together, potatoes and deadly nightshade, fig trees and oaks.

Similar fluidity is present in medicine's classifications. Ailments may be grouped according to how or why the information needs to be processed, by location of symptoms, their treatment, the threat they present to public health, their etiology, their prognosis, how much they cost to cure, and so on. The logical anatomical link between the common cold, asthma, and pulmonary tuberculosis would dissipate before a public health interest, where pulmonary tuberculosis would sit more clearly with salmonellosis (a gastrointestinal infection) or the plague as a notifiable disease.

For us to be able to classify a disease, it must first be visible to medicine. This visibility is not based simply on technology: being able to distinguish a particular microbe or genetic translocation. Rather, such recognition requires differentiation between the idiosyncratic and the generalizable. Do one person's fever and achy joints have anything to do with another's? If they don't, they're more likely to remain unfiled and unclassified: not a disease but an individual expression of something yet to be understood. The example of Lyme disease is helpful to understanding this question of visibility. Lyme disease was named in the mid-1970s. It was not hard to name and was easy to identify, as there was a clear infectious agent at the source of the disease with a specific vector, a tick-borne spirochete. Despite the tangibility and empirical evidence of its existence, it was not easily visible. The low-grade fever, headache, malaise, and joint pain of its sufferers could easily have been the result of any one of a number of systemic, infectious processes. However, the clustering of cases within a geographic region and in a particular time frame foregrounded this particular condition as a discrete, nameable entity worthy of research and for which a causative agent had to be sought. A number of Connecticut mothers (from the area around the town of Lyme) brought the cluster to the attention of public health officials. Had the cases been more geographically dispersed, the sufferers less articulate, or public health officers less receptive to its description as a unified condition, it might not have been named (Aronowitz 1998).

A diagnosis must not only be visible but also agreed on. There is a difference between presuming links between particular groups of symptoms and including the diagnosis in medical taxonomy. AIDS is a case in point. While we might have a clear picture of what AIDS is today—an acquired immune deficiency resulting from infection by the human immunodeficiency virus— it went through many previous configurations. Initially, it was the opportunistic infections typical of AIDS that were recognized. Clustered observations of pneumocystis carinii pneumonia and Kaposi sarcoma in particular populations (homosexual, hemophiliac, Haitian, and heroin users as well as those who entered into sexual relations with people from these groups) were considered as the disease problem. Many causative factors were evoked, including fungi, allergies, and chemicals. The isolation and identification of HIV and agreement on its contribution to the observed immunodeficit did not occur until 1984 (Gallo and Montagnier 2003).

Deciding what warrants grouping into categories and what needs to be seen as idiosyncratic and isolated—just one person's sickness—is part of how diagnosis organizes and directs medicine and public health (and is the challenge embodied in Ockham's razor). At an individual level, the clinician will classify the patient complaint, assessing symptoms for characteristics that bring to mind a particular pathology, a previous case, a textbook memory. Collectively, classification of diseases validates, locates, and distributes: designating whether a disease is real, if it is psychological or physical, under what subdisciplinary jurisdiction it falls, what treatment it requires, how many resources should be assigned to it, and so on.

Ultimately, the goal of classification is to simplify. Recognizing the similarity between conditions in order to group them provides a basis for communication, for logical connection, for research, and for statistical analysis. For a problem to be counted as a condition, it must first be identified as "the same as" or "different from" another; if different, the distinction between the two must be clear, or at least rational. As Arnold's "joints" illustrate, distinctions can be made in any one of a number of places. Zerubavel (1991) uses a contrasting metaphor, describing nature as a continuum broken up as we see fit. Both of these positions underline the fact that to classify is to reify. Diagnosis is the *making real* of conceptual categories.

Speaking of the "conceptualization" of disease is not to suggest that diseases do not exist. It is rather to point out *how* they come to exist. A disease might be conceptualized on the basis of its causation. For example, dengue fever is an infectious disease caused by one of four dengue viruses. It may result in bleeding disorders and a skin rash; despite these features, it is not conceptualized as either hematological or dermatological.

Disease conceptualization can be based on location (meningitis) or on symptoms (migraine). And diseases may be reconceptualized on the basis of new knowledge and understandings. The history of a blood disorder referred to in the nineteenth century as chlorosis, which subsequently went through numerous configurations on the basis of identity politics, laboratory techniques, and therapeutic approaches, confirms that there is no timelessness about disease and that technology cannot confirm all (Wailoo 1997).

In this chapter, I explore the aims of classification in general and their embodiment in medical diagnosis, using liberal historical examples of the diagnostic project. Classification schemas serve as archives of the practical politics of medicine (Blaxter 1978; P. Brown 1995; Bowker and Star 2000). From John Graunt's seventeenth-century *Reflections on the Weekly Bills of Mortality* to the tenth and still-current revision of the *International Statistical Classification of Diseases and Related Health Problems*, these nosologies highlight changes in medical models, legislation, and belief systems as much as they do the changes in medical knowledge. But mainly I will focus on why we classify in medicine: the rationale for splitting illness into different categories and the political and social compromises that these categories conceal.

The Aims of Classification

To classify is to arrange things in groups that are divided from one another by clear boundaries (Durkheim and Mauss 1903). Classification determines the response or reaction we should have in the presence of one group of objects (or conditions) as opposed to another (Hayes and Adams 2008). Seeking to understand classification and how it operates is not a new concern. Aristotle's doctrines of categories were the backbone of his philosophical inquiry. Aristotle presented a "schema of things" that accounted for both the particular and the universal (Novak 1965).

Aristotle's classification is hierarchical. The highest level on this hierarchy is the category, of which there are ten, including substance, quantity, quality, relatives, somewhere, sometime, being in a position, having, acting, and being acted on. The category contains a range of differentiated "species," which themselves may be further divided into genera. The point at which no further differentiation takes place is where the "particular" of a species finally sits at the lowest level. The category starts at the most general, branching progressively down to the lowest level, where the individual substances, such as "this man" or "that horse," are found (M. Cohen 2008).

Many centuries later, in 1837, William Farr echoed Aristotle's intent, couching the importance of the universal in scientific terms. He referred to classification as "a method of generalization" whose value was in its ability to serve as basis for empirical research, to "facilitate . . . inquiries and . . . yield general results" (qtd. in World Health Organization 1957, p. viii)

Classification theorists have postulated a number of aims of classification. These include (among other things) organizing knowledge (Jacob 1992); developing a useful description of a sample and discovering unsuspected but potentially important clusterings (Fleiss et al. 1971); achieving stable and predictive classes (Silvestri and Hill 1964); and perhaps above all, as Richardson wrote at the beginning of the last century, reducing a disorderly mass to an orderly whole (E. Richardson 1901).

Classifying is at the heart of how we understand the world. It is, according to Zerubavel (1991), the means by which we bestow meaning on things and concepts around us. It creates the "diagnostic niches" into which we place what we feel, see, smell, eat, and so forth. It is how we explain our experience of life and how we partition the social world.

Robert Sokal (1974) describes classification as having three aims. While his at-the-time novel approach to classification in the natural sciences (numerical taxonomy) was not universally accepted and has since been superseded by other methods, the aims he describes provide a succinct summary, useful for understanding disease classification. Reminiscent of Aristotle's desire to see the individual in the general, Sokal attributes to classification the following purposes: streamlining memory by grouping individual cases into representative groups; determining relationships between the members of one category and those of another; and generating questions about how the order that a classificatory system embodies has come to be. Classifications should help us to think about nature efficiently, he writes, explaining: "The world is full of single cases: single individuals of animal or plant species, single case histories of disease, single books, rocks or industrial concerns. By grouping numerous individual objects into a taxon the description of the taxon subsumes the individual descriptions of the objects contained within it" (p. 185).

Classification also seeks to create meaningful juxtapositions or interfaces between groups of objects. Classification can only be about isolated, bounded boxes if there is something beyond the boundary. It is part of a system in which one category sits in relation to what it isn't. The system makes generalizations about constituent objects feasible and meaningful, such that an object classified as X is not Y, or is mainly not Y and is more reasonably X. Nonidentical items may thus sit in same classificatory categories. For example, cows and people are both animals, despite having different numbers of legs, while cows and chairs, despite both having four legs, are unlikely to be found in the same category (Sokal 1974).

One final aim of classification is to be heuristic (Sokal 1974). A classification provides a hypothesis from which investigation into the perceived order can take place, be tested, and provide insight into etiological, social, and pragmatic explanations for the system of categorization. Systems to describe nature are dynamic; the best means for classifying objects (conditions) are constantly evolving as new explanatory frameworks, causative factors, and idiosyncratic presentations come to the fore.

Classification of Diseases

Classifying disease (diagnosis) has many intended purposes that serve both medical and lay interests. Some of these purposes serve both interests simultaneously, and others are more specifically linked with one group or the other. From providing a common language for discussing diseases to creating personal and collective identity, diagnostic classification organizes other activities beyond any immediate therapeutic goal. I review in the next few pages some of the primary goals of disease classification.

Clearly, diagnosis is the foundational step in determining the appropriate therapy for what ails an individual. Indeed, seeking treatment often leads the pursuit of diagnosis. By identifying the disease, one is a step closer to identifying a concordant treatment and cure. When cure is not available, at least a prognosis may often be agreed on. With a sense of what to expect from a particular condition—how things may progress—it may be easier to accept one's sort.

As Engelhardt (1992) writes, "One invests labor in making a diagnosis not simply in order to know truly, but because one would hope to be able to avoid or mitigate some unpleasant state of affairs. In the case of prognosis, one wants at least to be able to plan for likely unpleasant future developments" (p. 73).

When a condition is diagnosed, a different range of remedies becomes available. Think of the diagnosis of infertility. Looked at from a nonmedical perspective, it could be described simply as the state of unwanted childlessness (Becker and Nachtigall 1992). As a disease, on the other hand, it gains access to an entire new arsenal of potential remedies. It becomes worthy of medicine's attention and warrants medical solutions. Arguably, infertility is not a disease in the sense that it causes no physical distress to its sufferers. It is not accompanied by gastric upset or sore joints. It may make people suffer nonetheless, distressed by the undesirable social condition of unintended childlessness. But it can be diagnosed and treated. A range of infertility treatments including hormonal manipulation, acute monitoring of cervical or sperm function, and in vitro fertilization simultaneously redefine this social problem and replace its social solutions. As a nonmedical condition, unwanted childlessness is remedied in other ways. Changing aspirations (say, refocusing desire on other aspects of life) and adopting or fostering children are legitimate social approaches to resolving the distress. However, such actions are "are apparently viewed as more undesirable once a biomedical approach is initiated because they symbolize a dual failure: the failure to conceive and the failure to be cured" (Becker and Nachtigall 1992, p. 468).

Diagnosis also serves an important didactic and communicative role in medicine. This is in contrast to ancient medicine. Ancient Greek medicine, according to historian Ilza Veith, did not have a medical terminology. "So long as medical knowledge was restricted, a narrative descriptive style was used to evoke a picture of a disease, where nowadays one word, a simple disease name, would suffice" (Veith 1981, p. 221). Developing a nomenclature would lead to working therapy, which in turn would enable communication between doctors and allow medicine to be more efficient in its tasks (Fischer-

Homberger 1970). Thomas Sydenham is generally credited as being the father of classificatory medicine, committed to naming disease in order to advance the field by enabling communication between doctors and between doctors and students.

"All diseases then ought to be reduc'd to certain and determinate kinds, with the same exactness as we see it done by botanic writers in their treatises of plants," he wrote. His goal was "the improvement of physick" (Sydenham 1742, p. iv). Fisher-Homberger (1970) wrote that Sydenham, and his good friend John Locke, threw themselves at nosology in a kind of despair. Medicine was not terribly successful in its task, and resignation, laced with hope, about the state of the field prompted them to consider that by engaging in this systematic classification of disease types, they might find that medicine could make strides toward improving survival. "I am persuaded," wrote Sydenham (1742), "that there never will be any great and considerable advances made in the art of *healing*, till all hypotheses and mechanical reasoning are out of vogue, and till men are come about again to the antient method of experiment, and the common obvious reasoning entire from thence" (p. vii).

According to Fisher-Homberger (1970), "Two notions of beginners in medicine on the one hand and medicine herself as a beginner on the other tend to overlap. It is true that the nosological systems were designed to help medical students, but they were also to further medicine as a science, for as such it had still not progressed beyond its initial stages. For centuries it had kept going astray. Its language had become confused and unintelligible. There had to be a radically new approach to it. Nosology provided a possible new approach and its terminology provided the linguistic means to deal with it" (p. 400).

As recently as the mid-twentieth century, the limitations of the language of medicine were observed by Michael Balint (1964), who explained the need for better diagnostic terminology in psychiatry: "This want of a proper language is one reason for the unsatisfactory and often irritating lack of understanding between the general practitioner and the psychiatric consultant. We psychiatrists cannot yet give the general practitioners the badly needed set of technical terms which they could use confidently and which would help them to understand the deeper personality problems of their patients. For the time being our descriptions of pathological states are vague, complicated, long-winded, easily misunderstood when not backed by lengthy explanations" (p. 40).

Disease identification and naming has been an important part of psychiatry's professional project, as I illustrate in the pages to come. The development and revisions of the *Diagnostic and Statistical Manual of Mental Disorders* were to provide a uniform language to discuss mental illness and a transformation of diagnostic categories that enabled psychiatry to become more like its medical counterdisciplines, shifting psychotherapy away from the physicians, creating opportunities for clinical research, and favoring psychopharmacology (Mayes and Horwitz 2005).

Diagnosis continues to be at the heart of medical education, serving both as objective and as heuristic. Medical textbooks are organized around disease types, with physiology and biology introduced and explained via disease categories. Disease principles and specific diseases organize how medical students learn about the body.

Diagnosis enables research about disease. Research takes place when like can systematically be described as like, testing treatment efficacy empirically, making generalizations about disease patterns, and understanding causes of illness and death. The first disease classification document was devoted to this aim. In 1662, John Graunt published the *Natural and Political Observations . . . Made upon the Bills of Mortality*, an epidemiological document studying where and when particular groupings of causes of death could be found. Graunt's publication sought to predict disease trends. He had observed that people tended only to look at the bottom line ("the foot") of the weekly bills of mortality, namely, how many people died. He felt that much greater use could be made of this information to protect the population. The bills could predict the frequency and proportion of "sickly years," (p. 37) the relationship between "healthfull and frutifull seasons," the difference between "City and Country air, &c" (p. v). He made strong representation for a more detailed and standardized classification of causes of death, which would provide information about the diseases of the kingdom. While the plague figured prominently in social consciousness, Graunt argued that to understand its impact, it had to be carefully distinguished from other diseases that "forerun the plague a Year, two or three" (p. 34) and compounded the mortality statistics.

Graunt's work had no design on medical education; rather it was published to identify mortality trends and extrapolate either remedial or palliative measures to enhance survival. This analysis, clearly, sought a social frame. "The observations which I happened to make (for I designed them not) upon the Bills of Mortality, have fallen out to be both Political, and Natural, some concerning Trade, and Government, others concerning the Air, countries, Seasons, Fruitfulness, Health, Diseases, Longevety, and the proportions between the Sex, and Ages of Mankind" (p. vi).

Graunt wrote the above in 1662 as he presented his observations on the Bills of Mortality to Sir Robert Moray of the Privy Council to King James. This early classification of diseases presented arguments for the recording of "accompts of Burials, and Christenings [to be] kept universally, and now called for, and perused by Magistrate" (p. vii).

The contemporary *International Statistical Classification of Diseases and Causes of Death* (ICD), (which I discuss further in the following section) followed Graunt's tradition of attempting to understand the causes of death in order to summarize and describe trends in mortality that could help direct public health initiatives and policy. Diagnosis thus enables statistical analysis of disease and mortality by providing categorical units for synthesis. This type of analysis can extend, however, far beyond simply recording mortality trends. Being able to count illnesses as diagnostic units enables many different kinds of measurements. Medical record review, quality outcomes, financial expenditure, and risk assessments use diagnosis to assess, measure, and predict what factors lead to what diseases, what diseases cost how much, and what treatments results in what outcomes. Deciding how much to reimburse for particular kinds of care, where to concentrate public health efforts, who is at risk from what, and how particular communities, organizations, or professionals "rank" in terms of disease performance—all this relies on the diagnostic unit.

Similarly, the evidence-based practice (EBP) paradigm relies on diagnosis. Its fundamental premise is one of decision making based on the generalizability of scientific findings. The absence of diagnostic categories prevents the systematic appraisal of reliability that EBP requires. Grounded in epidemiological understandings of illness and therapeutic efficacy, EBP uses diagnoses and their associated signs, symptoms, and treatment as the specific targets for intervention and appraisal.

A clinical diagnosis, with its inherent biomedical justification, contributes to sickness identity, both individual and collective. Susan Sontag (1978) describes illness as the "night-side of life, a more onerous citizenship. Everyone who is born holds that citizenship, in the kingdom of the well and in the kingdom of the sick. Sooner or later each of us is obliged, at least for a spell, to identify ourselves as citizens of that other place" (p. 3). By recognizing the "other place," the newly diagnosed emerges from the isolation of his or her private disease, locating new networks of support, but also a transformed identity. The individual illness fits into a wider explanation that may include many other individuals with similar, or at least related, complaints. It also offers the potential for politicized collective illness identity (P. Brown et al. 2004).

Klawiter's work on breast cancer speaks eloquently to how diagnosis (specifically breast cancer) creates both individual and collective identity (Klawiter 1999). In the mid-1980s, cancer became a movement, with its advocates, its survivors, and its campaigns. By the early 1990s, breast cancer inspired a specific social movement of its own with a variety of politicized identities with which women variably identified. These identities were not uniform; Klawiter describes three. The first revolves around honor and survival. It casts medicine as the great white hope and early detection as an important arm in the battle to beat breast cancer. It is linked to normative femininity and courage. It uses fighting words and celebrates those who have vanquished the disease. She describes the pink-beribboned breast cancer survivor as "proudly, voluntarily, and publicly mark[ing] herself . . . visually embodying an identity not otherwise apparent. This is an act of social disobedience-a collective 'coming out,' a rejection of stigma and invisibility, and a simultaneous appropriation of the traditional color of femininity for the survivor identity" (Klawiter 1999, p. 111).

An alternative to this identity is one that mobilizes against biomedicine, emphasizing the inequalities inherent in the system and the biased focus on heteronormativity. It promotes activism and social services. Finally, a feminist environmental justice movement casts breast cancer as the result of a toxic global cancer industry with interests in promoting as therapeutic the carcinogenic chemicals that are at the root of the disease. In this case, the person who has breast cancer is a victim, fighting the pharmaceutical industry, whose focus is on profit, whatever the human cost.

The ability of the diagnosis to convey identity is powerful. The patient who refers to him- or herself as "diabetic" or "manic-depressive" incorporates the disease as part of the self via the syntactic construction of being: I *am* diabetic (Fleischman 1999). Becoming the diagnosis, being replaced by it, is reinforced by synecdoche (taking the part for the whole), common among the conversations of attendant health professionals. "Can you check on the MI [myocardial infarction] in room 3?" The patient, summed up as this disease or that body part, becomes subsumed by what was only part of who she or he was before (Fleischman 1999).

The transformative nature of the diagnostic moment may tell us we are sick even before we are ill and provides us with a clear message about who we are. Things will never be the same again: "In a person suffering severe or chronic illness, just as in a community suffering an epidemic, disease provokes a crisis of self definition; internal boundaries shift, and the complex structures of identity rearrange themselves" (Klinkenborg 1994, p. 78).

Certain diagnoses have mythic significance for the identity of their sufferers. Tuberculosis was held to selectively attack the romantic exile, the artist: both passionate and passive. It was considered a mark of breeding and of culture (Star and Bowker 1997). One nineteenth-century husband wrote of his wife, "She has that ardent pallor which we have always dreamt about and which devours our hearts. On her dull skin, light dances in a violet and greenish glow. Her teeth shine like those of a young tigress, and her eyes have a strange gleam which frightens me" (qtd. in Bricart 1985, pp. 182–83). Melancholy was similarly long held as a badge of honor, the mark of "all truly outstanding men with creative and moral qualities," according to Aristotle (qtd. in Melechi 2003, p. 13). The "melancholick" had a particularly elevated social status unlike the populace, who were more likely to be afflicted with mundane grief, or the mopes (Melechi 2003).

The multiple purposes of diagnostic classification—treatment and prognosis, medical education and communication, research, and identity—are enacted by the classification systems used by medicine and by the lay pursuit of diagnosis to organize the experience of illness. I briefly review two important diagnostic systems used in Western medicine, the ICD and the *Diagnostic and Statistical Manual of Mental Disorders* (DSM) before concluding this chapter with a commentary on how values and political actions become embedded in and reproduced by diagnostic classifications.

Classification Systems

Prominent contemporary disease classificatory documents such as the ICD and the DSM start with a historical genealogy, highlighting other statistical and nosological precedents. The influence of, and deference to, history is an interesting feature of contemporary medical classification. As Blaxter (1978) expounded, medical classifications are perhaps best considered as a "museum of past and present concepts of the nature of disease" (p. 10). Phil Brown (1995) adds that contemporary classification systems contain vestiges of many prior conceptions of disease, as distant as eighteenth-century botanical classification or later clinical pathology, as well as a number of other models, some no longer explicitly present in practice but still firmly engrained in the classification system.

Were disease more like library books, one could impose an external constraint on how and in which section conditions would be filed, and it would simply be a matter of allocating a particular condition to a given classification, creating a logical rationale for the cases of slightly looser fit. However, medicine has, according to Blaxter (1978), built its classification system by identifying its parts first before the whole, thus creating a structure that bears the indelible imprint of its antecedents.

This back-to-front approach to a system is not surprising, or even avoidable. Changes in medical theory, technological ability, or values are frequent enough that they cannot give rise to new classifications systems at each turning point. That such changes lead to remodeling rather than reconstruction is evident in the presence of named diagnoses that hark back to their historical origins (Blaxter 1978), such as Raynaud, Down, and Graves syndromes.

International Statistical Classification of Diseases and Related Health Problems

The ICD is a diagnostic classification system published by the World Health Organization (WHO). Its presence infiltrates medical bureaucracy if not medical practice. It is used to collect and compare morbidity and mortality statistics around the world. The ICD is part of a "suite" of classifications published by the WHO, including also *International Classification of Functioning, Disability and Health* and the *International Classification of Health Interventions*. All of these classification systems have been negotiated and approved by the WHO member countries and are used for international comparisons and reporting (Madden, Sykes, and Ustun 2007).

The ICD is what Bowker (1996) refers to as an "information infrastructure." It is embedded in myriad databases, supports medical work, has international reach, is learned as part of membership in the medical profession, and is linked with numerous conventions (p. 50). Its purpose and shape are grounded in an information-gathering practice that is defined by nations anxious to understand, support, and monitor their citizenry. What makes the ICD interesting as a medical classification document is its genesis in politics of the state. Classification is an important mechanism by which states may promote their political and economic functioning. Protecting the health and longevity of its citizens is central to the modern state (Bowker 1996, p. 52). The ICD was developed as a response to nineteenth-century epidemics, which themselves were only enabled by the modern imperialist who could get from here to there in a shortened span of time. This meant that the bacillus at the heart of an epidemic in one country could make it to another before its vector (the diseased individual) died, spreading diseases well beyond their previous frontiers (Bowker 1996).

To discuss these imperialistic microbes coherently across borders, classifications too had to be able to cross boundaries, a purpose that the ICD undertook to satisfy. However, the ICD has never been universally accepted or consistently applied. Some countries, particularly tropical ones, have maintained that their concerns are inadequately represented, while others have not had the infrastructure to implement its use (Bowker 1996). The Dutch developed a double system to manage their international obligation to reporting causes of death while maintaining the decorum required by the families in relation to stigmatizing diseases. Certain causes of death would be anonymously reported to the state (syphilis, diseases of the prostate, and suicide), while more palatable causes of death were provided on the death certificate given to the families (Bowker 1996).

From its precursor documents in the 1890s, which sought to track causes of death, to its tenth revision, currently in use, each edition of the ICD provides a description of its scope and function, which progressively increased to include a range of new uses. In 1909, the Bertillon classification (the classification previous to the ICD on which the latter is modeled) made clear its intent: "A statistical nomenclature of causes of death . . . has the . . . humble but practical goal of enabling statistical organizations to summarize the thousands of reports which are submitted to them in as truthful and as comparable a way as possible. Anything which would distance them from this goal should be discouraged" (Bertillon 1909, p. 7, translation mine). And further: "A statistical classification . . . should be . . . statistical and purely statistical" (p. 9, translation mine). Persisting in this view, the 1957 ICD specifies that the purpose of a statistical classification "is primarily to furnish quantitative data that will answer questions about groups of cases" (World Health Organization 1957, p. vii).

However, by the eighth revision of the ICD, it described new purposes, such as hospital indexing, as possible uses to be made of its classifications. The next revision expanded the functions of classification to include—beyond the statistical project—a health management role, supporting the indexing of "medical records, medical care review and ambulatory and other medical care programmes" (World Health Organization 1977, p. xv). Nonetheless, this document still distances itself from clinical classification, as "to describe the clinical picture of the patient, the codes must be more precise than those needed only for statistical groupings and trend analysis" (p. xv).

Contemporary nosology is not contained in one text or classification document. Modern doctors and medical students are faced with an array of resources. In the past, one (or perhaps several) general medical textbooks, with periodical updates, might have been placed prominently on the GP's shelves and consulted to help the clinician separate the fine crackle of acute bronchitis from the rhonchi of emphysema. Now, with the exponential expansion of medical information and improved means of information storage and display, Internet-based resources have assumed a dominant role in both medical education and clinical use, pushing paper resources aside (Bove 2008). The online environment provides an immediate range of diagnoses from which to choose. Commercial electronic products such as UpToDate and Diagnosaurus provide condensed literature reviews and recommendations for diagnosis and treatment.

The diagnostic process might not employ a unique standardized classification system, but the postdiagnosis process often includes classification. Read Codes, as one example, are the standard codes for use in primary care information systems for the UK National Health Service (Swayne 1993). Devised for use in computer systems, these codes are "intended to be comprehensive, including all that health care professionals, informal carers, and patients themselves may want to say about their situation, for any purpose" (p. 30). The Read Codes are used to achieve an impressive number of purposes, from health data collection to public planning, marketing strategy, insurance reimbursement, treatment protocols, and practice evaluation.

David Rothwell (1985) claimed that over 200 statistical systems in the United States alone coded health, occupational, and environmental conditions. Still today, these include such products as the Systemized Nomenclature of Medicine, which is a coding system with a controlled vocabulary and thesaurus; the Diagnosis-Related Groups, a classification that groups conditions on the basis of their expected resource use for fiscal purposes; the Medical Subject Headings thesaurus produced by the National Library of Medicine to enhance information retrieval; and of course, many others.

The explicit goals of classification are accompanied by implicit functions as well. None are perhaps as remarkable as the degree to which classification anchors professional status within medicine and legitimizes various branches of medicine. The ability to classify illness as true or feigned, medical or psychiatric, infectious or autoimmune distinguishes patient from doctor and establishes the authority of the medical profession. As Freidson postulates, diagnosis lends status to the doctor, whose task it is "to authoritatively label as illness what a complainant suspects to be illness, and also to label as illness what was not previously labelled at all, or what was labeled in some other fashion, under some other institution's jurisdiction" (1970, p. 261). Medical classifications also designate and validate the respective roles of subspecialists from within. Foucar (2001) adds that classifications "codify the interaction between contemporary sub-speciality politics and contemporary scientific classification tools" (p. s10). Classification has played a particularly pivotal role in defining both psychiatry's position relative to other medical specialties and dominant paradigms within the specialty.

Diagnostic and Statistical Manual of Mental Disorders

Psychiatry has always guarded the boundary between health and illness, deviance and disease (Rosenberg 2006). Those who have unusual or yet-to-be-understood physical illnesses may find their complaints explained as resulting from psychogenic causes. This tendency probably relates to the certainty that guides medicine and the difficulty that it has in gathering in behavioral or physiological outliers: a classificatory predicament. What do we do with the individual case, the idiosyncratic, the marginal or deviant that the agreed-on categories fail to accommodate? As we have seen in the preceding paragraphs, diagnosis seeks to generalize, but generalization is not always possible, and mental illness is frequently used as a residual, or "wastebasket," category into which those behaviors that defy other explanations must be filed. It is not unusual for physical diseases to be incorrectly attributed to psychiatric disorder either early in the disease history of an individual or in the history of the disease itself. Multiple sclerosis and Huntington disease have both been mistaken for psychosis or psychosomatic disorders (J. Stewart 1989; Skegg

1993). (See chapter 4 for more on the psychiatric explanation for medically unexplained symptoms.)

Mental illness was summarily classified in historical epidemiological texts. John Graunt (1662) made reference to "lunaticks," and to the "sort of mad-man who thinks to ease themselves of their pain by leaping into hell . . . [and] die in self-murder" (p. 21), but did not focus on the signs or explanations for these conditions. After all, his interest in disease was only concerned with whether or not it caused death. He didn't think there was much to classify. These cases, he wrote, the "generality of the word are pretty able to distinguish" (p. 13). He did acknowledge the chaos that was "Bedlam" (or Bethlem, an asylum run by the City of London from 1547). He could not differentiate in his accounts of causes of death those who died at Bedlam as a result of their madness or from other causes (p. 20).

There was little expansion in the classifications available for categorizing mental illness over the centuries, with only one category present in the U.S. census of 1840. It subsumed two conditions: "idiocy" and "insanity." In 1880, seven categories of mental illness became available for census takers (Gaines 1992). By 1918, the *Statistical Manual for the Use of Institutions of the Insane* expanded these categories to twenty-two (Kutchins and Kirk 1997).

How mental illnesses are defined, considered, shaped, recognized, studied, and revised by medicine today is captured in the successive versions of the DSM. In 1952, the American Psychiatric Association (APA) published the first version of the DSM under the auspices of the Mental Hospital Service. This publication reflected important shifts in psychiatric practice, privileging psychodynamic and psychoanalytic approaches, acknowledging the influence of environmental factors in mental illness, and making space to consider taxonomically a range of less severe forms of mental illness treated outside of the hospital (Kutchins and Kirk 1989). It was, however, a practical document, which sought to standardize nomenclature rather than define a field (Gaines 1992).

The DSM was a document that would be, and continues to be, revised. While the revisions are putative reflections of the advancement of medical (in this case, psychiatric) knowledge, they serve as valuable sociomedical archives for tracing beliefs, actions, power, and interests (P. Brown 1995). The first revision of the DSM took place in 1968 and represented a minor exercise in categorical alignment rather than the controversial conceptual and political modification that the DSMs were to become. The DSM-III revisions were motivated by three distinct forces, according to Kirk and Kutchins (1997): public protest over the medicalization of homosexuality, clinician dissatisfaction with available disease categories (and notably the need for precision in order to undertake pharmaceutical trials), and third-party payment of psychiatric care. Evidence of subspecialty politics is also clear in the DSM-III. Published in 1980, it exemplifies how revamping a classificatory system conveyed status and legitimacy to a languishing branch of medicine.

Psychiatry was marginalized within the medical community, its therapeutic roles subsumed by nonmedical professionals, its scope of practice restricted by those who funded care. Tensions within the field and a bourgeoning antipsychiatry movement led the psychiatric discipline to reconstruct psychiatric classification around symptom-based categorical diseases rather than etiologically defined entities (Mayes and Horwitz 2005). The new manual "transformed the little-used mental health manual into a biblical textbook specifically designed for scientific research, reimbursement compatibility, and by default, psychopharmacology" (p. 263).

DSM-III also sought to site mental illness within a medical model, gaining credibility through a more scientific, biological focus. Symptoms took on a different meaning; they became signs of disease rather than symbols of distress (Gaines 1992). The histories of subsequent revisions of the DSM (DSM-III-R and DSM-IV) highlight how the DSM is part of an always-ongoing scientific process that makes each edition provisional and every category dynamic. However, the goal of avoiding controversy and providing an illusion of professional consensus underpins the procedures that contribute to the DSM revisions. For example, the DSM-IV held as a working principle that no changes could be made to the previous document that did not have sound empirical foundations. As a similar criterion was not in place for the earlier version, the illusion of quality control resulted in concretizing classifications with little or no empirical grounding (Kutchins and Kirk 1997).

Currently under development as I draft these pages, the DSM-V promises to generate no less controversy or debate. Its draft diagnostic criteria were posted on the APA Web site in 2010 and were open for discussion until late April. New categories of disease, such as "psychosis risk syndrome" are creating angst among practitioners who argue that such diseases would result in very high false positives. Categorizing risk (more on this in chapter 6) widely expands the potential field of sufferers and opens the field to the overuse of antipsychotic medication, with its own risks and side effects (Frances 2010).

Kutchins and Kirk (1997) emphasize that the succeeding DSMs create an illusion of unified professional consensus, when in fact there is, they believe, widespread confusion, disagreement, and controversy. However, the DSM still shapes the profession, and the profession in turn cements the putative professional importance of the DSM. Academic psychiatrists anecdotally report that reviewers for psychiatric journals request the use of DSM categories over any other, including the ICD, reinforcing its importance as the bible of psychiatry.

The DSM's treatment of homosexuality is a poignant example both of how the DSM is an arbiter of diagnosis and of how controversy and political pressure shape its content. Homosexuality was listed in the DSM-II as a sexual deviation, in line with necrophilia, pedophilia, sexual sadism, and fetishism. During the early 1970s, a number of factors converged to influence its removal from the DSM. Kutchins and Kirk (Kirk and Kutchins 1992; Kutchins and Kirk 1997) detail the various changes both in the profession and in civil rights awareness that spurred the transformation of homosexuality as a diagnostic category. I summarize their discussion here.

Kirk and Kutchins's explanation for the removal of homosexuality from the DSM relates (inversely) to the disease discovery process that Phil Brown (1995) describes as the way by which new conditions find their expression in formalized disease classification. I discuss this model in greater depth in chapter 3. In brief, this discovery process includes lay discovery, social movement, and professional and institutional factors. While lay persons or groups might argue that a particular set of symptoms should legitimately be considered a discrete disease entity, their ability to achieve institutional recognition is usually contingent on sympathetic doctors or institutions supporting their position.

In the case of homosexuality, a reverse process took place. What was posited as disease was actually, many argued, a variation in the range of human sexualities, and its continued promotion as diagnosable opened the door to repressive and often violent actions on the bodies, minds, and rights of homosexual men and women. Individual actions, social movements, and professional and institutional factors all came to challenge, and ultimately alter, the place of homosexuality in the DSM. It should be made clear that changes in the status of this diagnosis were not made on the basis of new empirical or scientific evidence but on the basis of social factors.

There were three strong forces in play at the time the DSM-III was being developed (Kutchins and Kirk 1997). First, gay liberation, a rights-oriented movement, had gathered momentum, particularly in light of horrid repressive treatments used against gay men, and after the Stonewall riots. Second, there were changes in the way the profession was viewing its mission and place. Attempts were being made to eliminate psychoanalytic approaches from psychiatric practice, focusing less on the theoretical causation of illness and the private-practice-based discipline and more on a descriptive, research-oriented discipline that mirrored mainstream medicine. And third, Robert Spitzer, a researcher and former psychoanalyst committed to removing psychoanalytic influence from the DSM, saw the issue of homosexuality as one that needed to be addressed. He saw both his professional development and that of the field as being linked to a coherent diagnostic index, which required reevaluating the place of homosexuality.

It was with this context as a backdrop that vigorous protests against the classification of homosexuality as disease were staged by gay activists at the 1970 American Psychiatric Association conference. The Gay Psychiatric Association was created and assumed a discreet presence, and that robust debate and contestation ended in a proposal to delete homosexuality from the DSM, which the board of trustees of the APA voted to do in 1973 (Kutchins and Kirk 1997). The negotiation of this deletion was a political one driven by polemic, values, and consensus. It was a struggle that required skilled management of opposing views.

This process of disease declassification punctuates the assemblages and boundaries that circumscribe disease and the authority to label it. It demonstrates the dynamic social nature of the diagnosis and the diagnostic process. As the conversion of homosexuality from crime against morality to disease and then to nondisease illustrates, diagnoses are *not* prior, ontological entities but *social* categories that organize, direct, explain, and sometimes control our experience of health and illness. This reinforces Bowker and Star's depiction of classifications as invisible work practices, which structure (without revealing) all of the points of view that are contained in any classification document (1999).

Revealing Classificatory Politics in Diagnosis

Zerubavel (1996) is eloquent in his discussion of the social construction of difference and similarity. Once classification is established, we are inclined to think of the categories as natural, when in fact, he reminds us, nature is a continuum that is only divided into categories on the basis of our understanding and conventions. Understanding classification requires, he writes, a recognition of cognitive diversity among members of different thought communities.

Because of this, and despite its tidy and compartmentalized aims, classification of disease cannot be invariant and lawlike, nor can it ignore the social. For a condition to be classified as disease, there first must be some human recognition of its undesirability. There must also be a technical capacity to discern it. There must as well be a collective will to assimilate it into the ranks of diseases rather than in, say, those of the moral, the spiritual, or the idiosyncratic. Once a particular condition is established as a disease, it must be placed within the range of diseases. Where it should sit is a decision involving, yet again, technological, social, and political factors.

The management of the nosological boundary, the splitting or grouping of conditions into "different" or "like," is not transcendent. The boundary "becomes" rather than "is" the objective organization of medical practice that does important work. As Bowker and Star (1999) emphasize, classifications give voice to certain perspectives and silence others. The paragraphs that follow provide some examples of the selective work done by medical classification and illustrate the stakes at play.

Medicine, for example, unconsciously assigns to psychiatry temporary guardianship of boundaries between disease and health; misunderstood conditions are directed its way until their mechanisms are clarified and treatments identified (Rosenberg 2006). Conditions such as pellagra, paresis (Rosenberg 2006), multiple sclerosis (Skegg, Corwin, and Skegg 1988), and other medically unexplained symptoms are shuttled to psychiatry as a catchall discipline for that which medicine does not yet understand. (I explore this in greater depth in chapter 4.)

The psychiatric diagnosis finds little favor with the lay sufferer and results in contest and conflict. Locating the unexplained in psychiatry encourages patient resistance to stigmatizing based on assumptions linked to psychosomatic disorders (Dumit 2006). While the physical explanation for a symptom confers, in most cases, a lack of personal responsibility for its onset, a psychiatric one implies that the patient might have the ability to both control and reverse the physical symptoms, an interpretation that may seem impossible to the sufferer and that brings with it stigma and shame.

Expert consensus panels commonly lead the discussions around disease classification (Aronowitz 2001), exemplifying a transition to a "big science" approach to classification (Foucar 2001), where experts appointed by authoritative bodies evaluate the evidence of the condition and make recommendations. Such an approach does not normally include a lay voice, despite the importance of lay discovery in many yet-to-be-named and often contested diseases (P. Brown 2008; W. Scott 1990).

Consensus is, of course, a social process, as is membership in such panels. It, like any other social process, enables the promotion of some values and the extinction or backgrounding of others. By way of example, the International Consensus Development Conference on Female Sexual Dysfunction, whose authoritative professional status enables its recommendations to serve as mandates, was organized by the pharmaceutical industry and supported by grants from Eli Lilly, Pentech, Pfizer, Procter and Gamble, Schering-Lough, Solway Pharmaceuticals, TAP Pharmaceuticals, and Zonagen. Its statement was produced by 19 authors who acknowledged financial or other relationships with 24 listed pharmaceutical companies (more on this in chapter 5). The findings of this committee were that urgent investigation was required to develop new classifications and definitions of sexual dysfunction (Jutel 2010a; Moynihan 2003). This paper and its findings served as the justification for numerous subsequent research reports presenting tools designed to capture this asserted reality, proposing medications to treat the conditions, and urging immediate attention to them. The interests of the experts are embedded in the classifications, which, by their design, convey the statistical potency to justify and rejustify their existence.

Clarke and Casper (1996) write about the heterogeneity of the actors involved in classification. They argue that the Pap smear classification systems that have evolved and mutated over many years are evidence of a kind of boundary object. The boundary object, as described by Star and Griesemer (1989), is a classification that accommodates the problem of common representation in intersecting yet heterogeneous social worlds. Boundary objects have "different meanings in different social worlds but their structure is common enough to more than one world to make them recognizable, a means of translation" (p. 393). In principle, a boundary object enables communication and acknowledges a range of interests; it is an example of negotiated order.

That the boundaries of particular classificatory boxes should meander might be seen conveniently (albeit inappropriately) as an example of the progress of science marching ever closer to the truth of conditions. The classifications of overweight and obesity are useful examples of the shifting boundaries that should be probed in order to understand, as Clarke and Casper (1996) propose, "what counts as biomedical knowledge, for whom, and for what purposes" (p. 603).

Classification in medicine has long histories. These are dual and yet intersecting. With numbers and generalization driving one thread and clinical advancement driving the other, they have nonetheless some commonalities, and an ever-increasing tendency to substitute themselves for one another, with, notably, the statistical tradition encroaching firmly on clinical practice. This notion that numbers are more systematic than reports may underpin the drift of the ICD from a statistical to a clinical document. The World Health Organization Web site (2009) identifies the use of the ICD (eleventh revision in preparation) as a tool for epidemiological, health management, and now *clinical* purposes, certainly a change from the boundaries between statistics and clinical practice set in previous revisions.

We can see one important paradox that medicine faces with regard to classification. Just as Aristotle's classification attempted to find the general in the individual, so too does medicine seek to establish similarities through classification in order to promote population health, allocate resources, focus research, and so on. Medical practice, on the other hand, focuses on the idiosyncratic individual. "The scientific basis of medicine," writes Cassell (1991), "does not recognize nor provide a methodology to deal with such individual variations on the level of patient-doctor interactions" (p. 20). Patient narratives, and notably the narratives of the doctors who find themselves unexpectedly in the patient role, underline the uniqueness of the illness experience, which may be glossed over by medicine in its pursuit of generalization (Jutel 2010b).

Classification is not value free. The evidence-based practice movement (which encourages weight as a proxy measurement for activity and diet, for example) values measurement over patient report. It also marginalizes unstudied populations, such as, say, Cook Islanders or Tongans. Despite the absence of population-specific statistics, close to 70 percent of these islanders have a body mass index of $\geq$ 30 (World Health Organization 2009b), are identified as among the fattest populations in the word, and are not spared from the stigma associated with being "fat." (On antifat stigma, see Hebl and Xu 2001; Jutel 2008; Teachman and Brownell 2001; Puhl and Brownell 2003.)

Each and every classification engages some social perspectives and shuts down others, but once a classification is established it reproduces itself in an intuitive way that silences debate. In classifying, medicine takes a snippet of nature but often fails to recognize that the boundaries of that slice are socially agreed on according to the dictates, conventions, and abilities of the field rather than already existing objects waiting to be discovered.

Hacking (2001) explains that "the idea of nature has served as a way to disguise ideology, to appear to be perfectly neutral. No study of classification can escape the obligation to examine the roots of this idea . . . no study of the word 'natural' can fail to touch on that other great ideological word, 'real'" (p. 7). Hacking's discussion points to the fact that classification seeks a picture of an object, a "fixed target," that is true to nature. Understanding how medicine decides to see one thing as distinct from—or similar to—another can help both doctors and those who study the medical institution understand more about how medicine simultaneously approaches and distances itself from its goals of preventing suffering. It can also better reveal the uses that are made of diagnosis by nonmedical agents and how these interface (or not) with the necessary medical project of diagnostic classification.

CHAPTER TWO

Social Framing and Diagnosis

Corpulence and Fetal Death

A neighbor of mine used to encourage her daughters to eat up food they didn't like by saying "Look at Hanan! If you don't eat up, you'll get like her." And when one of them shouted, "I like Hanan! I want to be like her," her mother said, to shut her up, "But Hanan will live all by herself. She'll never have children and nobody will ever call her Mama." How could I carry a child? Would the fetus have room, or would it be squashed up against my pelvis? How would it get its nourishment, seeing that the food I ate didn't seem to put any flesh on me? HANAN AL-SHAYKH (1994)

Diagnosis is medicine's classification tool, and as we have seen, it cannot be considered in isolation from human deliberation and agency. Classification is a process that relies on the ability to distinguish same from different: clustering those things that resemble one another in a group, distancing those items that don't belong. The seemingly natural fit that explains medical categories is nonetheless linked to many social phenomena: what we are technically able to recognize as same or different and what differences we consider to be significant. One might think that the medical diagnosis is embedded with an extra degree of realness in contrast to other categories. Doesn't the evidence-based system in which medicine is practiced provide some natural proofs to underpin medical classification? There is, of course, a materiality to disease that, on some level, seems logically to repel social construction. Asthma, tuberculosis, and gout are all real in the sense that they have biological markers or clinical features that meet certain standards of evidence. Yet this evidence is not adequate to remove the medical diagnosis from its social frame. I am using the term "social frame" in the same way that Aronowitz (2008) does: as an alternative to "social construction," a term, he argued, that often carries with it confounding antimedical and cultural relativist baggage.

Social constructionism emerged as an attempt to break with a positivist approach that considered social facts as measurable entities (P. Brown 1995). The uniform social reality of positivism was replaced by the assumption that ideas are "constructed, negotiated, reformed, fashioned and organized by human beings in their efforts to make sense of the happenings of the world" (Sarbin and Kitsuse 1994, p. 3). Implicit in this approach is the idea that human beings are agents, not simply passive entities or disembodied intellects that possess information (Sarbin and Kitsuse 1994).

One of the most influential foundational works in social constructionism is Peter Berger and Thomas Luckmann's *Social Construction of Reality* (1966), in which they argue that reality, objectivity, and facts are the product of social interactions and appear to be external to individuals only because they are sustained by the practices of many people.

Social constructionism contains four key assumptions (Burr 1995). First, it is traditionally critical of taken-for-granted knowledge. It insists that we should be highly skeptical of the idea that observations of the world "unproblematically yield its nature" (p. 3). Knowledge is not, then, simply the reflection of some external reality. Second, social constructionism assumes that the ways we understand the world are historically and culturally specific. How we make sense of the world, the concepts and categories we use, are the product of our history and culture. Third, knowledge of reality is the product of interactions between people. It is through everyday interactions that people make sense of and compose the world around them. "Truth" is therefore the product of social processes involving negotiation between people (p. 4). Fourth, each kind of knowledge, which is produced through social negotiations, then brings about, or invites, different kinds of action. The way we make sense of the world therefore influences what sorts of actions we engage in and how we interact with others. Following these key tenets, social constructionists argue that the proper focus of inquiry is detailed examination of the social practices of people as they engage with each other.

A challenge presented to the sociologist of diagnosis by this approach is contained in the argument that social constructionism does not adequately address the tangible physical reality of illness. Best's "contextual constructionism" provides one way out. It gives credence to the empirical world, recognizing that the claims and categories and actions of people are in regard to "something" (Best 1993). The researcher should therefore also engage with this "something" to provide some sort of empirical verification to the social conditions that are being constructed. Phil Brown (1995) advocates an approach that is similar to this contextual constructionism. He postulates the importance of taking the physical reality seriously, while still emphasizing the importance of wider social forces and interactive decision making.

Aronowitz skirts the issue of how disease's tangible realities are entwined with social conceptualization by avoiding the term "constructionism" completely. "Social framing," he contends, dispenses with the idea that there are no physical realities and implies the systematic study of social forces in the categories and classifications of medicine.

Social framing is the way that societies "generally recognize, define, name and categorize disease states and attribute them to a cause or a set of causes" (Aronowitz 2008, p. 2). But social framing also shapes the reality of those at risk of or affected by the diseases in question. In this chapter I provide two vignettes depicting different medical diagnoses. Each diagnosis is, on one hand, indisputably documentable but on the other is strongly framed by, or in turn frames, social as well as biological reality. I have chosen to examine corpulence and fetal death in this light because of how observable they actually are. Unlike those diagnoses that are easy to debunk because their cultural content is so close to the surface, overweight and stillbirth mark unquestionable physical realities. While we might be able to contest what constitutes "chronic fatigue" or argue to what "normal" sexuality "hyposexual desire disorder" is juxtaposed, we can't argue the fact of a dead fetus. Similarly, fatness can be observed, pinched, prodded, and photographed. It is hard to refute that it is there. Even while there is no dispute about their existence as observable phenomena, these diagnoses are also socially negotiated categories. This is why I have chosen them as a heuristic for the principle of social framing and its place in medical classification.

First, I consider overweight as an example of a diagnosis that is strongly framed by beliefs about how the body's appearance is directly linked to both its moral and its physical core. I show how something as tangible as weight is still strongly associated with the social in its meaning and its presentation. Overweight is actually a new condition; it can be framed as a diagnosis only in a social context in which scales are available to determine body weight (in distinction to qualitative "fatness") and in which there is a prevailing confidence in the ability of statistical assessment of weight to assess individual health. I show how weight has become assimilated as a proxy measure of well-being in Western society, a practice that initially was strongly resisted and remains dubious.

Then I discuss the fraught diagnostic terms surrounding fetal death. The implications embodied in the terms "abortion," " stillbirth," and "miscarriage" establish conflicting subject positions for mother and fetus and have both legal and administrative consequences for the woman who fails to give birth to a live child. I have subtitled this chapter "Corpulence and Fetal Death" to punctuate the fact that these conditions can be just as easily seen in nonmedical as in medical terms.

Corpulence

In 1931, Jean Leray, consultant physician at Bride-les-Bains, wrote a textbook entitled *Embonpoint et obésité: Conceptions et thérapeutiques actuelles*. This was a book designed to present a complete technical picture of the pathology of adiposity and its remedies. Curiously, the word *embonpoint*, translated in English as "plumpness," comes from the expression "*en bon point*," or "in good condition." Overweight has not always been a disease, as this etymology confirms.

Is it possible to think that overweight was not always perceived as a health problem? Overweight is indeed a new disease, but not because people are fatter than they once were. Rather, overweight could not exist as a category of analysis before the twentieth century because, while scales existed, they were too expensive for doctors' offices or for personal use. As a result, weight was not a feature of obesity. This is not to say that fatness did not exist; it featured as a topic of study in both medical and lay circles for centuries. It was mentioned, for example, by Hippocrates. However, fatness and overweight are two distinct concepts, and it is this distinction that provides a key to the conceptualization of overweight as a disease. The words "fat" and "obesity" are qualitative descriptions of corpulence, but neither suggests measurement or the idea that there is some target weight ideal for good health. Nineteenth-century physicians viewed obesity in qualitative terms; Herrick (1889) called it an "increased bulk of the body, beyond what is sightly and healthy," and Thomas (1891) referred to it as "excessive development of the adipose tissue." Diagnosis of obesity was therefore unrelated to weight.

Today, on the other hand, obesity can be measured. The body mass index

(BMI), which I discuss below, calculates corpulence by a formula comparing the weight of the body to the square of its height. It's a technical, objective piece of science that doesn't require the patient to speak or the doctor to look. Weight is not only the diagnosing tool, but when there enough of it (and even the absence of what could be labeled obesity), it becomes a disease in and of itself. The World Health Organization (2003) refers to an "epidemic" of overweight. In the same way, the Centers for Disease Control (2005) lists overweight as a "disease or condition" and provides links to teaching documents that explain that the prevalence of overweight has increased to "epidemic proportions." Its existence as an object of epidemiological study confirms overweight as a disease rather than the simple descriptive adjective it used to be. Overweight and obesity are referred to in the same breath in texts of all kinds, insinuating overweight as a stepping-stone to the already well-established diagnosis of obesity.

What are some possible explanations for the emergence of overweight as a disease entity? Two important phenomena provide a strong foundation. The first is the importance accorded to measurement in understanding health and illness. The second is the strong emphasis that Western society places on normative appearance. These two factors are reinforced by the commercialization of self-management through the gym, diet, and pharmaceutical industries.

The Scales Don't Lie

Measurement of the body, including weight, emerged in the nineteenth century as part of a general endeavor to establish rules about the nature of mankind and of subgroups within the species. The BMI, used today to determine overweight and obesity, was devised by Adolphe Quételet (1870) and was motivated by the religious incentive of discovering the presence of God's rules on earth.

Body measurement was the focus of anthropometry, anthropology, phrenology, and physiognomy even before the nineteenth century. Determining character, criminality, mental illness, and racial purity on the basis of size of different body parts was a particular preoccupation of the scientific community. Lavater (1855) generated a massive catalog assigning personality traits to physical signs. Similarly, Lombroso and Ferrero (1895), in their work comparing the body types of prostitutes, female lunatics, and "normal" females, wrote of measurements: "We would retain them as the frame, so to speak, of the picture; or, rather, as the symbol, the flag of a school in whose armoury numbers furnish the most effective weapon; and we would recommend such retention the more, that whenever a difference does result on measurement, the importance of the anomaly is doubled" (p. 2).

Using measurement for the assessment of physical health, however, was not as prevalent. Dr. Jean Leray, in his 1931 analysis of plumpness and obesity, devoted a number of pages to the different formulas and tables purporting to identify the perfect healthy weight but reduced their importance to "theoretical interest" and chose rather to accept Leven's definition of safe body weight as a person's "average weight, maintained over a number of years, as long as the subject has been well" (p. 7, my translation). Leray argued that the correct weight for an individual could not be determined by standardized tables. Similarly, William Christie (1927) warned readers that "no weight table is sufficient by itself to base an estimate of the ideal state." He continued: "Standard tables which show the average for men and women of our race at any given age and height are fallacious, because no allowance is made for the distinctions of personal physique, nor consideration given to obvious rolls of fat" (p. 23).

But it did not take long before most physicians capitulated to the ease of use and purported objectivity of scales in the assessment of patient health. This may have been in part due to a change in the cost, availability, and size of scales. At the end of the nineteenth century, the *Lancet* (1897) spoke of the presence of scales in the doctor's consulting room, presenting the "Reliance Weighing Machine" in its "Notes and Short Comment" section. The journal commented that "hitherto, these personal weighing machines have taken up too much room in a consulting room and the expense has been too great" (p. 1316). Later, advertisements for these scales asserted that they were a "useful adjunct to the consulting room" (New inventions 1899, p. 940). Undoubtedly, as scales became more available and as concepts of evidence in medicine were afforded more primacy, weight became an important part of the doctor's assessment.

Hillel Schwartz (1986) argues that "the body when weighed told the truth about the self. Once gluttony had been linked to fatness and fatness to heaviness, heaviness had still to be regularly identified by numbers on a scale, rather than by vague and subjective sensations" (p. 147). Doctors would be relieved to have a straightforward mechanism for judging patient health that did not rely on patient reports of eating or exercise habits, or what Leray referred to as "wellness." The scales wouldn't lie, while the patient might. As Foucault (1963) wrote in his history of the clinic, the medical gaze saw the patient as a barrier to the truth: "In order to know the truth of the pathological fact, the doctor must abstract the patient . . . [T]he medical gaze . . . [addresses] all that which is visible in illness, but starting from the patient, who hides that which is visible by showing it" (p. 8, my translation). In the clinical assessment, the patient's story can obstruct the clinician's pursuit of the facts of the illness.

Scales for weighing a patient would become part of the trend (described in Rosenberg 2002) toward "instruments of precision" that emerged in the late nineteenth century. These apparatuses, including microscopes, thermometers, and later manometers, radiology equipment, and electrocardiogram machines, offered objective mechanisms for capturing, standardizing, and monitoring disease. Rosenberg argues that being able to express results in standardized units enabled disease to be "operationally understood and described. It was measured in units, represented in the visible forms of curves or continuous tracings" (p. 244). This standardization and measurability form the basis of contemporary diagnosis, epidemiology, and evidence-based medicine, which produce and reproduce overweight as a disease entity.

An important tenet of evidence-based medicine is that scientific research informs clinical decisions and therapeutic approaches. Good medicine, in evidence-based practice, is that in which the clinician, using sound judgment and experience, artfully interprets the findings of research studies (which themselves attempt to minimize variables, bias, and researcher conflict of interest while testing for the generalizability of the findings) and applies it to her or his patient. But such integration is possible only in the context of standardization, where variability can be defined, populations discerned, results compared, and similarity to the patient established. Implicit therefore in the research-based or experimental model is the quantification of cause and effect and the measurement of, and focus on, in this case, body weight.

With the ability to quantify corpulence comes the potential to track its distribution, prevalence, and correlates. In turn, this allows a description of normality and a delineation of the bounds of normal build, which subsequently naturalizes concepts of difference and deviance. Numbers imply neutrality, as qualitative researchers who have long fought for recognition precisely because of the nonquantitative nature of their studies would report.

Yet even as scales became a standard feature of medical rooms and a range of weight classification systems became both available and implemented, the social shaping of diagnostic options continued to vary. From 1942 to 2000, no fewer than eighteen different ideal, desirable, normal, suggested, acceptable or other categorical formulations for weight were implemented by a range of official classificatory documents (Kuczmarski and Flegal 2000). A weight considered "ideal" in 1942 (say, 5′7″ and 162 lb. [170 cm and 73 kg]) would have been "desirable" in 1959, "acceptable" in 1985, and "overweight" in 2000.

Today, the current gold standard for weight assessment in the Western world is the BMI. However, it too is a moving target. Since 1990, the upper limit of healthy weights has changed from 27.8 kg/m² to 24.9 kg/m², and the cutoff range for healthy weight on the basis of age and gender has been modified (Kuczmarski and Flegal 2000). Changes to the classification system are due to increasing scientific input relative to risks and benefits of particular classificatory groupings. Yet such science cannot be assumed to be either universally accepted or unproblematic. The Dietary Guidelines Advisory Committee (1995) reports that mortality increases above a BMI of 25 kg/m² and recommends that this be considered the lower limit of a risk category. In contrast, Flegal et al. (2005), using data from the National Health and Nutrition Examination Survey and on the basis of the estimated relative risk for mortality of BMI categories, report that overweight (> 24.9 kg/m²) is not associated with excess mortality. Similarly, Orpana et al. (2009), in a study of more than 11,000 adults, find that mortality is actually *lower* in the overweight and in class 1 obesity (BMI 30–34.9).

These challenges, and others like them, to weight as a marker of wellness have not managed to unseat the scales as primary tool in the creation of the diagnosis of overweight. They continue to dictate wellness and create a convenient mechanism for understanding corpulence, one that reflects the anxiety of a society concerned with normative standards of appearance.

Normative Appearance and Health

The importance of appearance in Western culture is the second cornerstone to the emergence of the framing of overweight as a medical diagnosis. While measurement underpins the creation of this condition, before it can be measured, it must occur to people that it is a concern: something that *should* be measured systematically and in the absence of complaint by the subject. We don't, for example, assess the length of the second toe as a routine part of health care, despite its being pathognomonic of Morton foot syndrome, unless the individual complains of metatarsal discomfort.

The visible presence of corpulence is pivotal in the privileging of weight as something that needs to be monitored. One's appearance, and how closely it matches normative expectations, are of great importance in Western society. Whether the standard of beauty is one of plumpness or of thinness, it is the departure from the standard that will be a source of concern embodied in social institutions, including, but not restricted to, the medical establishment, the church, and legal and educational fraternities. Not only has beauty been associated with goodness and ugliness with vice, particular forms and presentations of the human body have been associated with various meanings.

Historical attitudes toward appearance demonstrate how deviation from physical norms is problematized, condemned, and, today, diagnosed. Early Christian doctrine uses metaphors of beauty to speak of virtue, with the "spotless mirror" (*speculum sine macula*) representing the goodness of the Virgin Mary and blemishes bearing witness to sin. In the fourth century Saint Augustine described the Holy Scriptures as a mirror that reflects the truth about the self. He wrote, "You're ugly, you see yourself ugly. But when you come in front of it in your ugliness and see yourself ugly, don't blame the mirror. Go back to yourself. The mirror isn't deceiving you, take care you don't deceive yourself" (Augustine 1990, p. 336).

Throughout seventeenth- and eighteenth-century texts, the appearance, particularly of a woman, was purported to reveal the inner nature of the individual. Wealthy Renaissance families used portraits of their daughters to arrange marriages, and these were required to convey as much information as possible about the individual portrayed (D. Brown 2001). Female beauty signified morality and virtue as well as membership in a particular social class. Closely linked in Renaissance thought and art, beauty and virtue were further highlighted by mottoes and emblems on the reverse of the portraits, punctuating the meaning portrayed by the primary image. The back of Leonardo da Vinci's portrait *Ginevra de' Benci* interprets the meaning of the portrait with the inscription "Beauty Adorns Virtue" (D. Brown 2001).

While it is not the purpose of this chapter to develop a discussion on the unequal focus of beauty as, in particular, a testimony to female virtue, it is clear that these discourses tend to target women. A highly developed notion of feminine duty is prevalent in texts from many eras and reflected in the contemporary media. These texts contain strong messages about a woman's individual responsibility to achieve the normative standards of beauty.

However, the idea that inner nature is revealed by external appearance takes a different form in the nineteenth century, as virtue became embedded in the discourse on health maintenance. While virtue once inscribed itself on the body in the form of beauty, the new virtue was good health, which can also be discerned by the appearance of an individual. In 1896, Ayer advocated its sarsaparilla as a blood cleanser: "Beauty begins in the blood" read its advertising, noting that "Beauty is blood deep, not 'skin deep'" (Ayer's Sarsaparilla 1896, p. 115), while the California Fig Syrup Company (1896) reminded readers that "one of the greatest factors in producing a clear, clean skin and therefore a perfect complexion, is the use of Syrup of Figs." And the Pabst Brewing Company (1897) spoke of a young mother "flushed with perfect health" after consuming its malt extract, the "best" tonic.

Mirroring the nineteenth-century description of health as a state of beauty, today we treat health as an esthetic state that we can assess through the shape and measurement of the body. Carole Spitzack (1990) describes health as a standard for attractiveness that heightens concerns about outward appearance in an imprisoning manner. "An aesthetics of health," she states, "not only requires slenderness . . . but appropriate skin coloring, muscle conditioning, facial structure, and an absence of facial lines or 'defective' features" (p. 36).

Art historian Barbara Stafford and ethicists John Puma and David Schiedermayer (1989) discuss the hidden role of visual and perceptual preferences in medical judgments about the abnormal (p. 214). There is a standard of homogeneity, they write, that governs how medical professionals respond to patients, how the law protects patient rights, and what defines our medical priorities. Normality, the dreaded bugaboo to which we aspire in cultural practices is, not surprisingly, just as deeply ingrained in medicine: "The unstated perceptual norm that governs our reactions to patients is predicated on a symmetrical and minimalist conception of beauty. Less is more. Even wins over odd. Homogeneity is better than complexity" (p. 214). Historically, however, physiology, ethics, and esthetics have attempted, and continue to attempt, to capture the symmetry of beauty or of good taste in measurement and geometry. Perfection by number and by form had, and continues to have, implications for the notion of what it means to be human and what it means to be healthy, reinforcing the esthetic of health described by Spitzack.

Being Overweight, Being Diseased?

Clearly, overweight is both a cultural and a medical concern in contemporary society. Vigorous gym, diet, and pharmaceutical industries pin their operations on the anxiety of those able to pay to strive for the perfect body. Helping people to consider themselves ill or at risk of illness provides a platform for piggybacking commercial interests onto medical authority. And creating a disease category out of a self-identifiable statistical deviation such as weight enables the commercial exploitation of those so afflicted. Self-assessment tools generate significant consumer interest (McEntee 2003). Those conditions that can easily be diagnosed by a consumer without medical intervention are particularly attractive to industry. For example, BMI calculators are popular features on pharmaceutical Web sites, such as those for the weight-loss drug Xenical (Xenical-Orlistat 2010) or the laxative Metamucil (Procter and Gamble 2009).

But the weight-loss industry extends well beyond the pharmaceutical companies and plays an important role in the generation and promulgation of the diagnosis of overweight. A large number of industries stand to benefit from the belief that overweight is a disease. This results in significant lobbying and product promotion based on the disease label (Oliver 2006). Weight reduction, muscle tone, and body shape are exceptionally strong markers of "health" to consumers (Spitzack 1990). The gym, diet, self-help, cosmetic, pharmaceutical, and many other industries have a financial stake in ensuring that people see their weight as problematic from a medical point of view (Jutel and Buetow 2007).

Peter Conrad (2005) refers to commercial interests as an important vehicle for medicalization. Examples of an implied medical endorsement for products and services are prevalent in advertising strategies, particularly in what Dixon and Banwell (2004) refer to as a "diets-making complex," or a vehicle, often exploitative, for the dominance of health considerations in all facets of dietary discourse. Transferring such information to the consumer implies a recognition of lay knowledge of health risk, buttressed by authoritative medical discourse and language that draw the individual into a closed circle of virtuous consumers who focus on important evidence-based truths.

Other researchers question whether the medical concern with overweight is a dangerous case of diagnosing nondisease. Physiologist Glenn Gaesser (1999) explains that the bulk of epidemiological evidence fails to support the "lose weight–live longer paradigm," and argues that contemporary medicine disregards the protective effects of moderate overweight with respect to osteoporosis, mortality, diseases of the lung, and some forms of cancer. A number of studies have reported that thinness and weight reduction can present a higher risk of mortality than obesity.

Gaesser points out that many independent factors covary with BMI, and teasing out those factors is a challenge. Lifestyle, exercise, and diet can affect weight and can also affect mortality and morbidity. Weight becomes a symptom rather than a cause but nonetheless is generally taken as a purveyor of truth in the context of evidence-based medicine. While an individual's account of activity level or dietary intake may be unreliable, BMI is purportedly free of bias. I use the word "purportedly" intentionally, for while numbers may appear free of bias, the meanings they capture are not benign. Standards for "healthy" BMI may apply to a population but say nothing about the health of an individual patient. Such standards do not even specify the population to which they are applicable. As such, they may not be relevant to certain peoples. Furthermore, BMI is a crude measure of body fat and ill suited to measuring health in certain groups (K. Robinson et al. 2005). Recent studies have cast doubt on the validity of BMI to represent adiposity accurately and on its ability to differentiate between populations (Nevill et al. 2006).

On this subject, one should note that BMI marginalizes unstudied populations, such as, for example, Cook Islanders or Niueans. Despite the absence of population-specific statistics, close to 70 percent of these islanders have BMIs of) 30 (World Health Organization 2009b). They are identified as among the fattest populations in the word and are not spared the stigma associated with being "fat." (On antifat stigma, see Hebl and Xu 2001; Jutel 2008; Teachman and Brownell 2001; Puhl and Brownell 2003.) The remoteness and small size of their populations exclude them from mainstream epidemiological study, making generalizations about the relationship between BMI and population health unreliable.

That overweight should be a disease entity is not a surprise given the beliefs on which Western approaches to the body are buttressed. What is salient, as Rosenberg (2002) notes, is that diagnosis poses a number of intractable social dilemmas and particularly the "difficulty inherent in fitting idiosyncratic human beings into constructed and constricting ideal-typical patterns" (p. 251). As Cassell (1991) points out, the effect of science on clinical medicine is considerable. Science's purported neutrality—its objective generalizations about populations and about diseases, and its reduction of the human condition into physiochemical terms—is at odds with clinical practice. Science is about generalization, while clinical assessment is about the individual.

The social framing of overweight as a diagnosis reflects the social reality of those who are overweight. The putative disease contains the possibility of both self-diagnosis and self-treatment. With scales and the wide-ranging availability of diet, exercise, and over-the-counter pharmaceutical products, there are far-reaching implications for reinforcing values about normative weight and also for creating unrealistic standards and expectations that fill hapless large people with feelings of inadequacy and guilt.

Fetal Death

Just as observable and "real" as plumpness, the death of a fetus in utero is an undebatable event. It can be seen, measured, recorded, studied, and compared. However, this does not remove it from a social frame with regard to its label or to its impact. Medicine provides a range of diagnostic terms to describe death in utero, each with different consequences for the women and families affected by the event.

None of these terms is value free; they embody a number of assumptions and beliefs about pregnancy, the mother, and the fetus. The words are part of a greater cultural and political context in which the end of any pregnancy takes place, a context that is fraught with challenges. The debates raging in the context of pro-life or pro-choice camps frame any unexpectedly terminated pregnancy. Does the not-yet-born baby/fetus have an autonomous existence? Does the woman provide a hostile or nurturing "environment"?[1] These discussions infiltrate the classifications of pregnancies that do not end in live birth. In the upcoming pages, I explore how the diagnoses of fetal death convey social values, affect social practices, and reinforce a number of conflicts that rage around pregnancy.

Giving a name or a diagnosis to a condition or, in the case of fetal death, an event, will always reflect the state of knowledge of the medical community at the time of the naming. As we have observed previously, that knowledge is strongly influenced by the values and concerns of the society in which the diagnosticians practice. We will see how such values infuse the diagnoses of fetal death.

The cultural content of the terms *abortion, stillbirth*, and *miscarriage* presents challenges. On the surface, these terms have simple meanings. The stillbirth is distinguished from the miscarriage and the abortion by the potential viability of the fetus. *Stillbirth* refers to the delivery of those infants who would have been viable on the basis of gestation at the time they left the womb but who emerge inanimate, differentiating them from the miscarried or prematurely aborted fetus/baby. In New Zealand, the Births, Deaths and Marriages Registration Act 1995 provides for the recording of information relating to births and other vital records. It defines "'still-born child' as a dead fetus that: a) weighed 400g or more when it issued from its mother; or b) issued from its mother after the 20th week of pregnancy." Other Western countries have similar definitions of *stillbirth*, some using both weight and gestation as defining characteristics, others using just gestation. For the purpose of establishing international comparisons, the World Health Organization (2003) recommends the recording of all deaths that take place in the perinatal period. This, according to the ICD-10, "commences at 22 completed weeks (154 days) of gestation (the time when birth weight is normally 500g), and ends seven completed days after birth."

Defining the event by gestation is not straightforward, particularly when organizations use different gestational cutoff dates. Different countries, and even different states or regional authorities within the same countries, use a variety of parameters to label stillbirth, leading to a lack of clarity and precision in the diagnosis. Developed countries generally use earlier cutoff dates than underdeveloped ones (Lawn et al. 2009).

Stillbirth implies potential viability that was thwarted by the pathological event. Yet viability doesn't fully justify the gestational definition. I should point out that what constitutes viability, like BMI, is not fixed. The state of knowledge of the medical community in a particular situation and at a particular time will determine whether or not it can maintain an infant born before term. This means that *when* and *where* a stillbirth takes place will determine what degree of prematurity is potentially viable. Think again of isolated island nations with limited life-support technology. Viability is thus not an absolute but is dependent on availability of resources.

This question of what gestation might reasonably reflect viability brings to mind recollections from my own nursing training in the early 1980s, when I helped look after a twenty-eight-week premature infant, born tragically to a mother in shock after her other children perished in a house fire. The staff looked on the child with horror as a "failed miscarriage," and many privately shuddered, thinking about the ethics of maintaining such a premature baby. Today, of course, infants of this gestation are regularly nurtured to maturity, a testimony to advances in the ability of the medical community to rescue premature infants. Perhaps to accommodate the fact that intensive care standards change over time and the fact that a premature infant who is not considered viable today may be tomorrow, the current definition of *stillbirth* also includes infants who, at twenty-one weeks' gestation, would be unlikely to survive if born alive today. And herein resides the challenge: if some currently nonviable fetuses are included in the definition of *stillbirth*, why aren't others?

The paradox arises from the fact that the diagnosis assigned to the pregnancy that does not result in a live birth confers a contradictory sense of order. Some nonviable infants may be considered stillborn, while others are not. The families of stillborn infants, even those outside the current limits of viability, are provided ritual outlets for acknowledgment of the conception and for grief, such as certificates of birth and death, burial, and gravestone, while those of late-term miscarriages are not—despite, in many cases, feeling the loss just as acutely.

Maintaining a lower limit for the definition of *stillbirth* may be due in part to the legalization of voluntary abortion based on gestational criteria. The implication of viability contained in *stillbirth* would be problematic for an aborted fetus, as it allows the rapprochement of abortion with infanticide. Emphasizing the ability of the fetus to live outside the womb is a prominent tool in the pro-life, antiabortion discourse. This autonomy is also ostensibly embodied in the miscarriage/stillbirth distinction, even in the absence of voluntary abortion. The terms themselves enforce this: *miscarriage* implies the failure of the mother/womb to protect the dependent fetus, while *stillbirth* conveys the potential of autonomous (albeit, temporarily supported) existence and the innocence of the mother in the fetal death.[2]

Rosalind Petchesky (1987) argues that fetal autonomy is reinforced by the use of imaging techniques, notably in pro-life propaganda campaigns. The ultrasound image of the baby/fetus shows it in isolation from the pregnant woman, recasting it as an autonomous subject and reducing the pregnant woman, at the very most, to the passive mediator of fetal growth. Petchesky reports how the images reinforce the absence of the pregnant woman, "representing the fetus as primary and autonomous, the women as absent or peripheral" (p. 268). This results in a climate where the woman can be cast as being in an adversarial position vis-à-vis her pregnancy. According to Kathryn Conrad (2001), the pro-life movement actively promotes this position through the maintenance of fetal autonomy, identifying an array of behaviors of the pregnant woman as risky and irresponsible, and positing the womb as a potentially hostile environment. The baby is depicted in its intrauterine environment, moving, breathing, and sucking its thumb. This endearing and powerful imagery emulates the family photo while erasing the woman from the frame. These images become an effective tool in the campaign to discourage voluntary abortion, as they cast the fetus as child and the invisible womb as "the most dangerous place in the world to be" (Ruth Riddick, qtd. in K. Conrad 2001, p. 159).

It is precisely whether the woman is attempting to give birth or to terminate the gestation that determines the individual meaning associated with the diagnosis assigned to the outcome of the pregnancy. The challenge to health care providers occurs when there is a mismatch between cultural and individual interpretations of where autonomy and agency reside in the birthing process. I next review the terminology used to qualify fetal death, its importance in the assessment of care, its impact on administrative processes, and the threats it may present to those who experience pregnancy loss or termination.

The infant mortality rate is often used as an indicator of national health. Discrepancies between nations and between different populations of the same nation are identified as major challenges to be tackled and constitute important priorities. Perinatal mortality specifically, including stillbirth and early neonatal death, is considered the measuring tool of a maternity service's performance (Health Funding Authority 1999). This focus is undoubtedly reinforced by the symbolic importance of conception, pregnancy, and infancy in Western culture. At no other time in life is the human existence so dependent on the concerted care of other human beings. At this stage in human development, one can easily witness the effect of human agency on health. In the absence of human intervention, survival itself is uncertain. This establishes the importance of care, and of health care in particular.

In midwifery practice, for example, stillbirth is an important measure of failure. Cultural conventions, deeply historical in origin, continually remind the midwife of the potential for the baby to perish. The modern title of the memoirs of eighteenth-century Frisian midwife Catharina Schrader is suitably extracted from a message of relief contained in her own records: "Mother and child were saved" (Schrader 1987). Contemporary conventions around the reporting of births also remind the midwife of this ominous threat. Conventional notes by the midwife adhere to the following formula: "XX hours: spontaneous vaginal birth, *live*, female, APGARS X and Y, etc." (emphasis added).

Documentation of obstetric history, birth notification, and hospital/home-birth databases contain side-by-side columns or choices for "live" or "stillborn." The New Zealand Midwifery Standards Review data sheet includes stillbirth as one measure of performance, clearly linking the professional development process of the midwife to the stillbirths of babies for women under her care (New Zealand College of Midwives 2004). Stillbirth is also commonly one of the measurements of quality in comparing outcomes of midwifery-led care and shared or obstetrician-led care, as in the famous randomized controlled trials carried out in Australia and in Sweden (Rowley et al. 1995; Waldenstrom and Turnbull 1998).

If stillbirth is a marker of professional performance, then we have to differentiate those deliveries that could never, in our contemporary setting, have resulted in a live birth (less than 21 weeks) from those that might have. The prospect of a pregnancy that could have resulted in live birth but did not strikes terror in the heart of a midwife or obstetrician. The impact of being involved in a delivery that unexpectedly does not result in live birth is horrifying. As reported by Cowan and Wainwright (2001): "It does not take much to rekindle the vivid nightmares of that experience and to relive the acid adrenaline nausea of impending disaster that overwhelm . . . [the midwife]" (p. 313). The emotional experience of the caregiver, be it a midwife or an obstetrician, will be subordinated to the grief of the parents and will often be assaulted by litigation, marginalization, and professional scrutiny.

If, on the other hand, the delivery could never have resulted in a live birth because of the short term of the pregnancy, the consequences for the caregiver are different. Self-doubt and terror evaporate with the disassociation from any potential guilt. The experience of a nonviable delivery would be referred to colloquially as a "miscarriage" and would be considered unfortunate but not tragic. Within the medical community, the formal description of such an outcome is "abortion." In contrast with the popular use of this term, which signifies *deliberate* termination of pregnancy, the medical meaning simply implies termination, with a range of adjectives to qualify the nature of the termination: voluntary, incomplete, spontaneous, threatened, legal, illegal, or recurrent. Curiously, the legal definition of *abortion* is quite different from the medical one. While the etymology is from the Latin *aboriri*, or "to miscarry" (*ab*, "away from," plus *oriri*, "to be born"), in New Zealand, the Crimes Act 1961 defines abortion in terms of intentionality: the "procurement of miscarriage," in line with, and reinforcing, lay definitions of the term—signifying intention on the part of the parturient and lending to confusion as a result of the liability inherent in the term.

Whether a baby's death is a miscarriage, a stillbirth, or an abortion will have not only legal but also fiscal and cultural implications. As Wilfred Mills (1977) pointed out in the *Lancet* many years ago, the distinction between an abortion and a neonatal death has significant social consequences: "A neonatal death will carry a birth and death certificate and thus an entitlement to a financial maternity benefit that would be lost if the event were classed as a late abortion."[3] This holds true today. Work and Income New Zealand, the source of welfare support in New Zealand, will only award a funeral grant for infants who were either initially live or who fit the statutory definition of *stillborn* (Ministry of Social Development 2003).

Similarly, the New Zealand Births, Deaths, and Marriage Registration Act does not accord personhood to a baby who is miscarried rather than stillborn. According to the interpretation of the act, *child* includes a stillborn child, while *miscarriage* refers to the "issue from its mother . . . of a dead fetus." While the bearer of either is considered a mother, she is only entitled to refer to her "child" if it meets a statutory requirement of 21 weeks' gestation or 400 g weight.

This statutory principle presents challenges. Midwives recall the difficulties encountered less than two decades ago if a multiple birth took place before the then-statutory definition of viability at 28 weeks. One twin might not survive birth, while another might live but die later. The existence of the twin who does not survive birth is not acknowledged in the same way as the one who does: in contrast to his or her sibling, the stillborn baby cannot be registered. Breathing outside the womb, rather than gestation, confers the status of child. With the renewed definition of stillbirth resting on 21 weeks' gestation, one might presume that this problem is resolved, but with the technical advances in neonatal intensive care, babies are resuscitated and saved at increasingly early gestational stages.

Not all peoples use viability or gestation in their assessment of personhood. The indigenous people of New Zealand, the Māori, have a different perspective on prebirth. Māori practices do not use gestational age as a distinguishing category, calling the preborn child *pepi*—the same name used for a child after its birth—regardless of its developmental stage. The *pepi* also has agency and decides to inhabit or to leave the womb. The cultural approach to the death of the *pepi* would not be affected by its gestational age either but would be constrained nonetheless by New Zealand statutory definitions. A *pepi* not considered a child under the Births, Deaths, and Marriages Act because of early gestational age can only be buried on the *urupā*, the traditional Māori burial place (Russell 2005) and in no other cemetery. Death before breathing is a prominent feature of Polynesian stories of creation, with Maui, the iconic Māori demigod hero, having left his mother's womb *pepi mate*, or stillborn, to be rescued by Tangaroa (god of the seas) and raised by Tamanuikiterangi (Erlbeck 2001).

In European culture, on the other hand, the difference between stillbirth and miscarriage entailed, and continues to entail, other legal consequences beyond death registration and legal burial. Unmarried women who lost their babies were subject to suspicion that they might have killed the baby to avoid the infamy of bringing an illegitimate child into the word. While a miscarriage was unfortunate, a stillbirth suggested at least the possibility that the mother had killed her infant. European women suspected of infanticide in the eighteenth century described their miscarriage as the delivery of "only blood" or of a substance "like a lump of flesh," thus denying the existence of a baby and placing the event in the realm of a "false conception" rather than a birth marred by infant death (M. Jackson 1996).

One might see parallels here with the recent case of "Baby Aaron," the much-reported discovery of a stillborn child in the sewage system of Hastings, New Zealand (One News 2005a). While there was no doubt, according to the coroner's report, that the child was born dead, the mother still risked charge and prosecution. Disposing of a dead baby is a violation of section 181 of the Crimes Act, which states that "everyone is liable to imprisonment for a term not exceeding 2 years who disposes of the dead body of any child in any manner with intent to conceal the fact of its birth, whether the child died before, or during, or after birth." The law does not define what constitutes a child, but it is clear that how the term is used is of fundamental importance. If the event is a stillbirth, the woman may be charged with a crime, while if it is a miscarriage, she will not be called to account.

Since "Baby Aaron" was discovered to be the fetus of a young unmarried teen (One News 2005b), one could speculate that its flushing away was evidence of the girl's denial of its personhood and also perhaps a gesture to preserve her own reputation. In this case, the construction of the event as birth or nonbirth and the fetus as child or nonchild has far-reaching legal and personal consequences.

While some continuity in practices surrounding the early termination of pregnancy might be present, representations of miscarriage vary according to the era in which it occurs. Leslie Reagan (2003) argues that today's pregnancy-loss movement draws on both the current antiabortion and feminist movements to comprehend and define miscarriage, female emotion, and motherhood. She also maintains that attitudes toward miscarriage have changed. In the twentieth century, miscarriage has variably been seen as a hazard, a blessing, or a tragedy, depending on its place in time.

The challenge presented by the issues surrounding a pregnancy that does not result in a live birth leads to the paradox of conflicting maternal subjectivities. Articulating fetal personhood imposes simultaneously on the mother the burden of guilt and the responsibility of care (depending on the birth outcome and the mother's participation in its achievement). This fetocentric model of pregnancy may also result in the removal of maternal subjectivity. On the other hand, denying fetal personhood denies maternity by creating the childless mother. Importantly, the values embodied in the terminology used within New Zealand texts can be at odds with the experiences of individual women. Petchesky (1987) points out a similar mismatch in women's views of fetal ultrasound images. Although the woman would seemingly be disempowered by removing her from the picture, thus treating her as a maternal environment without agency, the ways women experience these images are not necessarily negative. The woman's response is always contingent on her individual circumstances—mainly on whether she wishes to be pregnant or not. For one woman, these images are an unproblematic first peek at a soon-to-emerge baby; for another, the images are an instrument of intimidation, creating a female subject, otherwise effaced by medical imaging technology, who is morally deficient and dangerous.

Likewise, the manner in which fetal death will be received by women, their partners, families, support systems, and health professionals depends on complex individual social and psychological circumstances. While one group might experience gestational death as loss, another might see it as relief—and indeed could voluntarily provoke it. It is the subject positions available to any woman who has experienced the gestational death of her child that are problematic. And yet neither the women nor any other individuals have the ability to change the diagnoses, the statutes, the laws, and the welfare benefits that reinforce these awkward positions. The value content of the language cannot simply be eradicated or modified to suit the circumstance, and the impact of the diagnostic category on death benefits, legal responsibility, and social recognition are considerable.

Health care professionals who attend pregnancies that do not result in the birth of a live infant cannot ignore the values contained in the diagnosis or, particularly, the conflicting potential impact on the women and their partners who have experienced this event as a "death" in the womb. At one level, it's obvious: despite the innocuousness of the term within the medical community, a midwife, nurse, or obstetrician would carefully avoid making reference to "spontaneous abortion" in the face of a grieving woman who had wanted to carry her infant to term. The connotation of this phrase among the lay population is simply too powerful to be ignored.

Frame and Be Framed

The very real conditions of corpulence and fetal death take root as they become actualized as medical diagnoses. The authority of medicine gives substance to their existence in different ways than if they remained outside its jurisdiction. The doctor rules on the fetal gestation, acting as a catalyst for legal, economic, and social events.

With respect to fetal death, medicine's authority first to pronounce what constitutes viability in gestational terms and second to reckon the gestation is contingent on cultural and technological factors. The same holds true for corpulence. As we look at current medically sanctioned ideal weights, we see paradoxical contradictions that are somehow trumped by the medical truths that seem to be based in something other than science.

Paul Campos and his colleagues (2006) doubt the putative obesity epidemic is the public health crisis it is cast to be by public health authorities and the media. They refute the fact that there is evidence of an epidemic. The changes in population weight are subtle, with a slight trend upward, hardly evidence of dramatic change in population health. Further, the increasing rates of BMI are not contributing to increased risk of mortality; general life expectancy continues to increase, with the lowest morbidity and mortality in so-called overweight categories. Statistical linkages between overweight and mortality are flawed, with inadequate control of factors such as exercise, diet, and demographics. Cardiovascular risk factors have also dropped in all weight categories (Flegal 2006). What justifies this focus on obesity if the epidemiology doesn't support the argument?

Campos et al. (2006) posit that this is a moral panic rather than a health crisis. Moral panics are "typical during times of rapid social change and involve an exaggeration or fabrication of risks, the use of disaster analogies, and the projection of societal anxieties onto a stigmatized group or an episode" (p. 58). Cast by the mass media as a threat to social values and interests, the moral panic is supported by "right thinking people." It is an event that is monitored and validated by socially accredited experts (S. Cohen 1980, p. 9). The notion of moral panic has been applied to a range of episodes: drug taking, crime waves, terrorism, and perhaps overweight.

Considering how the alleged obesity epidemic fits the criteria of a moral panic helps to critique the classification of overweight as a disease. While use of the word *epidemic* may be only metaphorical, it conveys an urgency previously reserved for the plague, tuberculosis, or other major infectious events. In the traditional epidemic, rapid containment is vital to the survival or at least the well-being of the community. With events such as the gradual rise in population BMI, the threat takes an extremely different form. The clichéd use of the word *epidemic* is linked to specific rhetorical and policy goals and has dramaturgic aims (Rosenberg 1992). "The intent is clear enough: to clothe certain undesirable yet blandly tolerated social phenomena in the emotional urgency associated with a 'real' epidemic" (p. 280).

In the case of the obesity epidemic, the language used is one of exigency. Obesity is seen as a threat to be fought, an insidious danger.[4] Understanding the urgency of this message and the reasons for which a language of epidemic and doom are proposed to describe the problems of obesity force us to consider the question of deviance. Deviance, in all cases, is attributed rather than inherent (P. Conrad and Schneider 1980). It can exist only in the presence of a grouping of subjects. That is to say one can be deviant only in relation *to* someone or *from* something else. Being corpulent in isolation is not deviant, and indeed is, or has been, normative in some settings and eras.

There are a range of definitional questions that should be asked by a student of deviance: "Why does a particular rule, the infraction of which constitutes deviance, exist at all? What are the processes and procedures involved in identifying someone as a deviant and applying the rule to him? What are the effects and consequences of this application, both for society and the individual?"(S. Cohen 1980, p. 13).

The rules in the case of obesity, and in its definition as deviant, are shaped by overlapping and conflicting fiscal interests. I have noted the financial gains to be made in the promotion, control, regulation, and treatment of obesity. But the interests may be other than financial. The Centers for Disease Control, for example, uses the threat of the obesity epidemic as an arm in the battle for increased funding for its policy initiatives and authority (Campos et al. 2006).

Diagnoses do capture reality, but the nature of that reality is fluid, situated, and social. Mirowsky and Ross (1989) compare diagnoses to constellations in the sky, made up of stars that are truly present but whose meaning comes from how we assemble them in recognizable patterns. The process by which a diagnosis emerges involves human—and by extension, social—discernment with all its accompanying baggage: technological, political, and cultural. A collective cultural position determines which symptoms we will see, which we will brush off as insignificant, how we make sense of what is there, and what social consequences the diagnosis will convey.

In both corpulence and fetal death, the lay perspective may be at odds with or disregarded by the medical diagnosis. Classification of "overweight" does not consider diet, exercise patterns, or even adiposity. Similarly, "spontaneous first-term abortion" does not capture the feelings a pregnant woman experiences at what she may consider to be the death of her son or daughter. Hunter (1991) describes how the lay and medical explanations can be at odds. The "transformed and medicalized narrative may be alien to the patient: strange depersonalized, unlived and unlivable. Returned to the patient in this alien form the medical narrative is all but unrecognizable as a version of the patient's story—and all but useless as an explanation of the patient's experience" (p. 13). The medical diagnosis does not consider how the individual has actually lived or explained and accounted for his or her condition and cannot necessarily be incorporated into his or her personal narrative.

This medical-lay discordance is at the base of the next chapter, which explores how diagnosis sits at the heart of the lay-professional encounter, both as a justification for consultation and as a source of potential collaboration, possibly leading to a cure but also to a contest.

CHAPTER THREE

What's Wrong with Me?

Diagnosis and the Patient-Doctor Relationship

> I jumped up and shook hands with this man who'd just given me
> something no one else on earth had ever given me
> I may have even thanked him habit being so strong
> RAYMOND CARVER (1998)

Hippocrates wrote that "if [the doctor] is able to tell his patients when he visits them not only about their past and present symptoms, but also to tell them what is going to happen, as well as to fill in the details they have omitted, he will increase his reputation as a medical practitioner and people will have no qualms in putting themselves under his care" (1983, p. 170). His words underline the important role of diagnosis in confirming the professional status of the doctor and in delineating the doctor-patient relationship. Diagnosis is at the heart of both, providing a rationale for the consultation, confirming the authority and prestige of the medical profession, and delegating the responsibility for labeling an illness.

The diagnostic moment is crucial to the patient-doctor relationship, as demonstrated by Raymond Carver's poignant, autobiographical epigraph to this chapter. The poem demonstrates how his own emotions and those of the doctor overlap and feed off each other, as he effaces himself before the doctor. Both submissive and generous, he holds back on causing unnecessary distress by reflecting his own pain back on the doctor while he endures this life-altering moment. Despite Carver's concern for the doctor's feelings, the doctor and

patient sit in different positions in this encounter—framed by diagnosis—
while nonetheless sharing its impact. The differences are grounded in perspective, education, experience, identity, emotion, and more. In this chapter,
I explore some of these differences and their consequences. I begin with the
illness and disease dichotomy, which describes how the matter of "not feeling well" becomes part of a medical narrative with diagnosis at its core. Then
we see how the authority afforded medicine grants it the right to determine
the narrative of illness and its subsequent management. Finally, I discuss the
changing roles of lay person and health professional in the diagnostic encounter and envision the potential this has for the study of health and illness
identities in the twenty-first century.

Illness and Disease

Pursuit of diagnosis brings patient and doctor together. Feeling unwell is
the usual prompt for seeking medical attention. And it involves a premedical
assessment in which the individual attributes his or her unwellness to what
he or she thinks is likely to be a disease rather than an external or nonmedical factor. But it is the inability of the lay person to fully interpret the situation, despite assigning it to the realm of the medical, that leads to the clinical
encounter (Leder 1990). He or she seeks the explanatory power of the diagnosis, which the doctor is authorized to deliver.

The lay person's desire to understand the discomfort—the cough, the rash,
the swelling, or the cramp—prompts an encounter with her doctor. The
process by which the illness is described in the consultation, in which the
complaint is described and contextualized, is the first step in "organizing"
an illness (Balint 1964). Balint's model of patient-doctor interaction sees the
patient's pursuit of medical opinion as an organizational task. This model remains relevant to contemporary lay-professional relations. Indeed, this model
may have even more pertinence in the era of the increasing patient autonomy
and knowledge. The patient consults the doctor to present an organizing explanation of his or her ailments for confirmation. In a sense, she "proposes"
a diagnosis.

Balint puts great emphasis on the diagnosis. The most pressing and immediate problem for the patient is *"the request for the name of the illness, for
a diagnosis. It is only [then] that the patient asks for therapy"* (p. 25). The
illness proposal must be recognized and negotiated with the doctor. This in-

teraction might take the form of a presentation of a symptoms. Already, the first step in organization has taken place. "I have a headache. Do you think it might be a tumor?" enables the doctor to organize the information gathering. Why do you think it might be a tumor? What is the nature of the pain? Have you any changes in your visual fields? The doctor ideally proceeds to a sequence of steps that rule in or out (in order of seriousness) the possible explanatory diagnoses, from brain tumor to migraine, stress, or benign headache. In the ideal encounter, or series of encounters, the doctor responds to the illness as offered, exploring the patient's organizational strategy, testing its pathophysiological coherence, offering alternative diagnoses until both patient and doctor can agree on the fundamental diagnosis underpinning the patient complaint.

Diagnosis is the medical reading of these symptoms: interpreting and organizing them according to models and patterns recognized by the profession. Leder (1990) describes this process as a "clinical hermeneutic" or interpretive project. The individual initiates an encounter with the doctor to obtain an explanatory position from which to approach the illness.

The distinction between illness and disease is important to the sociology of diagnosis. This differentiation was not made clear in earlier sociological texts. Freidson (1970), for example, used the terms interchangeably. Today, however, the distinction contains important conceptual differences that inform discussions of diagnosis. Illness is the personal experience of sickness (Kleinman, Eisenberg, and Good 1978). Illness problems are those that result from undesirable changes in social or personal function. How an individual perceives these problems, explains or labels them, and seeks remedy originates from a cultural context. This in turn influences the decision to access, or the response to, medical services. In any case, as Locker (1981) points out, to consider oneself ill is to presume a biological cause for a disvalued state of being.

Disease, in contrast, is framed by the biological rather than the personal. This is not to say that it is bereft of cultural content, rather that it represents what Western medicine considers biological or psychophysiological dysfunction (Kleinman, Eisenberg, and Good 1978). Fleishmann (1999) refers to diseases as conceptual entities, or "categories of clinical taxonomy . . . extrapolated from an aggregate of similar illnesses on the basis of what is thought to be common to the illnesses so classified" (p. 7). Disease is diagnosed, illness is not; rather, it is presented to a clinician as *presumed* disease. The transformation from illness to disease takes place through the intermediary of the doctor and the diagnosis.

While not all illnesses can be diagnosed, their narratives are the starting point for diagnosis. Note that there is more than one narrative: the patient's and the doctor's stories juxtapose and merge for a diagnosis to materialize. The patient's stories, emerging from his or her own experience, culture, and consideration of the role of the doctor, are transformed into medical accounts upon their telling. The doctor interrogates, interprets, and retells the story, establishing the "plot" and a diagnostic organization (Hunter 1991). In Leder's model, the patient has already determined that the explanation for his or her discomfort is medical in nature and that it is a doctor (rather than a different social authority, say a rabbi or a lawyer) who will confer meaning to the narrative. Illness is the story that results when an individual sees the interpretation in terms of health and medicine. In contrast, diagnosis is the story of medicine, told in the language of disease. "In the narrow biological terms of the biomedical model," says Kleinman (1988), "this means that disease is reconfigured *only* as an alteration in biological structure or functioning" (pp. 5–6).

Arthur Frank (1995) claims that a social expectation of being ill is not just seeking care but "a *narrative surrender*" in which the patient's story is relinquished to the doctor's, which is told through diagnosis and is "the one against which others are ultimately judged true or false, useful or not" (pp. 5–6). Kleinman maintains that doctors are taught to be skeptical of patients' narratives about illness, a view shared by Foucault (1963), who wrote that clinical medicine sought unequivocally to silence the patient, "who, ". . . by trying to show things, ends up concealing them" (p. 8, translation mine).

The diagnosis thus confers legitimacy to illness yet does not necessarily align with the patient's narrative for a number of reasons, not the least of which is the position from which the stories are recounted. Illness narratives "reveal what life is like for the narrator . . . [including] the practical consequences of managing symptoms, reduced mobility and so on. In telling their story, individuals also reveal, or indeed may assert, their self and social identity" (Nettleton et al. 2004, p. 49). Medical narratives come from an institutional position, which presumes the absence of the lived experience. It is the objectivity of scientific classification (in this case, the diagnosis) that confers authority to the label. Diagnosis is the fulcrum of the medical narrative. The judgment that this infers, as Frank asserts, may deny the self and social identity that the story of illness embodies.

Frank refers to illness as the experience of living through disease. It begins, he writes, "when popular experience is overtaken by technical expertise, including complex organizations of treatment. Folk no longer go to bed and die, cared for by family members. . . . [They] go to paid professionals who reinterpret their pains as symptoms, using a specialized language that is unfamiliar and overwhelming" (1995, p. 5).

The languages of disease and illness may be peculiarly discordant. "A transformed and medicalized narrative may be alien to the patient: strange, depersonalized, unlived and unlivable. Returned to the patient in this alien form the medical narrative is all but unrecognizable as a version of the patient's story—and all but useless as an explanation of the patient's experience" (Hunter 1991, p. 13). Such alienation occurs when the medical model takes inadequate account of the illness problems (such as how the patient has actually lived, explained, and accounted for her dysfunction) and is unable to incorporate this in its own narrative via the diagnostic label.

Blaxter (2009) movingly describes her personal trajectory of illness and the means by which the process of diagnosis effaced her lived experience of disease. Diagnostic technology replaced her own voice as the focus of medical attention. Symptoms and patient history were subordinated to scan results; patient knowledge and information, even clinical examination, took a backseat. In Blaxter's experience, the abnormal PET scan result could be explained as a "shadow" from her youth, possibly a vestige of a childhood tuberculosis—an explanation refuted rather hastily by her lung specialist.

The degree to which personal and professional narratives align may contribute to health outcomes, but it also illustrates the degree to which the diagnostic moment is framed by medical authority. Enabling a patient story—its plot, characters, setting, and description (rather than inserting the patient's words into a clinical picture)—acknowledges the patient's expertise in the construction of illness. It allows "joint authorship" by doctor and patient of the explanatory framework, the therapeutic decision, and the clinical outcomes (Clark and Mishler 1992).

Medical Authority

Diagnoses and their classificatory systems are an important collective arrangement that defines and enables the influence of professional medicine. But at an individual level, the ability to assign the diagnosis confers power to the doctor as allocator of resources (De Swaan 1989). The diagnosis legitimizes sickness. As discussed previously, when a doctor deems a patient's condition to be medical, the latter receives previously unauthorized privileges such as permission to be absent from work, priority parking, insurance benefits, reimbursement for treatment, or access to services. The doctor certifies the medical nature of the complaint and "medical advice" informs administrative and policy decisions.

Authority in medicine comes from its ability to define and delineate behaviors, persons, and conditions, write Peter Conrad and Joseph Schneider (1980), but also from the organization and structure of the medical profession. Medicine has an officially approved monopoly over the right to define health and to treat illness, which results in its high public esteem (Freidson 1970). The doctor, as the agent of medicine, is accorded a prominent position in the hierarchy of expertise and a mandate to exercise his or her authority over that of other health professionals and lay people (Freidson 1970).

The medical dominance articulated by Freidson is not, however, immutable. In 1988, Light and Levine argued that the power of the medical profession was already in decline, as evidenced by the introduction of malpractice lawsuits, profit-driven administration of physician performance, and cost-management strategies in medicine. More recent evidence of change in the status of doctors is present, according to Lupton (1997a), in increasing patient complaints, increasing use of alternative therapies, critical media portrayals of doctors, and lack of financial autonomy. Further, wider access to information has led to changes in the doctor-patient relationship, with patients more willing to challenge their doctor, dispute findings, or seek advice outside of the doctor-patient relationship (Lupton 1997a). Doctors are not alone today in the authority to diagnose. A range of other professionals, including chiropractors, nurse practitioners, and physiotherapists may diagnose certain conditions in some countries.

The patient-doctor relationship was historically one of an authoritative, paternalistic manager of care with a submissive, patient[1] recipient. In 1939, G. Canby Robinson described the relation of doctor and patient as unique. He explained: "The natural authority of the doctor, the confidence the patient feels in his professional knowledge, his unselfish, disinterested respect for intimate communications, the tradition, so long accepted, that the relationship between doctor and patient is confidential and the sentiment of the patient that the more the doctor knows about him, the more helpful he can be, all these attitudes and assumptions establish a basis for free and unbiased communication that is possible in few other human situations" (p. 2).

This relationship resulted, in part, from an imbalance in knowledge. The circulation of information about pathophysiology and normal biophysical function was limited to particular professional and scientific circles. In 1958, for example, Pratt, Seligmann, and Reader noted low levels of patient participation in doctor-patient interactions. They attributed this to patients' having little understanding of their diseases and their etiologies and treatments. Patients neither expected nor requested information from their physicians. In turn, the physicians acknowledged the patients' lack of medical knowledge, viewing such ignorance as a liability in terms of patient compliance, or likelihood to accept and follow the doctor's interpretation, explanation, and recommended treatment of disease. This is an example of a paternalistic interaction, where the patient is like a child, who submits him or herself to the guardianship of a kind and compassionate physician (Emanuel and Emanuel 1992). Patient autonomy is contained in assent and is subordinate to the beneficence of the physician.

Changing Roles in Diagnosis

Yet recently there have been assaults on the diagnostic role of medicine. These come from all angles. Lay social movements advocate for diagnosis and recognition of conditions often refuted by the medical institution (P. Brown and Zavestoski 2004). Avid commercial forces have been eager to tap the modern patient's increased access to previously privileged medical information, seeing in self-diagnosis an excellent avenue by which to promote particular conditions and, by extension, their concordant therapies (Healy 2006). But health policies too have encouraged a transformation of traditional relationships in health care, emphasizing a more active role for the lay person, whose expertise is derived from experience rather than knowledge (Wilson 2001).

Seeking other avenues for diagnosis is not a new phenomenon, for, just as

Hippocrates described the importance of the medical diagnosis, so too did he describe the unruly patient, reluctant to submit to medical care. He questioned their resolve: "Although they have no wish to die, they have not the courage to be patient." He wrote, "Is it not more likely that they will disobey their doctors rather than that the doctors . . . will prescribe the wrong remedies?" (Hippocrates 1983, p. 142). He emphasized the knowledge gap between lay person and doctor: "The symptoms which patients with internal diseases describe to their physicians are based on guesses about a possible cause rather than knowledge about it. If they knew what caused their sickness, they would know how to prevent it" (p. 145).

Today, however, lay people are far more likely to have specialized information about what causes their illness than in Hippocrates's time. Clinical decision making has changed its locus, according to Nettleton (2004). The lay person who consults the health care professional is no longer the submissive and compliant "patient" but an expert partner who brings his or her experience of illness to the differentially specialized medical practitioner. Medical knowledge has escaped ("e-scaped," in Nettleton's phrase), flowing as information through myriad electronic networks and Internet sources, enabling the patient to access and interpret information about disease well before her encounter with the doctor. Access to formal medical information is no longer confined within or controlled by medical institutions. Data from the Health Information National Trends survey in the United States confirmed that only 10.9 percent of U.S. adults go to their physicians first for health information, with almost half using Internet resources as their first source of information (Hesse et al. 2005).

The power of the physician is reduced by the availability of medical knowledge outside of the halls of learning, which creates an "informed consumer," rather than an acquiescent patient, who enters the clinical encounter with a different agenda than in the situation described by Pratt and colleagues. The relationship is no longer a one-way power-dependency relationship but an encounter based on knowledge (albeit unequal) about health and disease. Previously, the relationship was an archetypal professional relationship in which the patient would approach the clinician for his or her field of knowledge. Now educated consumers may consult the physician for support in making choices about information they possess in advance of the encounter. Emanuel and Emanuel (1992) would refer to this as the "informative model," in which the objective of the clinical encounter is for the physician to elucidate the options available to the patient, thus enabling her to make an autonomous choice.

Transforming the place of medical authority is not without challenges. Positioning patients as consumers opens the door for them to become the vulnerable prey of disease mongers. Indeed the ability to assess quality, reliability, and morality of health information is not necessarily within the grasp of most lay people, presenting a difficulty on two fronts. On one hand, any attempt to mediate access to information or to recapture control of its delivery will infringe on lay autonomy, returning the patient to the paternalistic care of the omniscient physician. On the other, consuming information without adequate understanding puts the patient, the doctor, and the doctor-patient relationship at risk. This is most evident in self-diagnosis, which can overturn traditional diagnostic responsibilities.

Self-diagnosis serves as an important tool in public health. Pandemic management during recent influenza outbreaks seeks to reduce spread of the influenza virus by asking people to stay away from the doctor if they have "the flu." The principle is that self-isolation is linked with self-diagnosis; the germs can stay at home. However, self-diagnosis is widely used by both commercial and lay disease-awareness campaigns, encouraging individuals to self-identify with a particular disorder and bypass the conventional diagnostic processes. The campaigns prompt the lay person to recognize signs of particular disorders and bring them to her doctor's attention. The advertising refrain "Ask your doctor if X [substitute name of remedy] is right for you" will be familiar to most North American readers. Both forms of self-diagnosis present challenges to medicine as they redefine roles in the doctor-patient relationship.

Patient safety is at the fore in medical literature reviews of self-diagnosis. A prominent theme in medical articles is that patients (having inadequate training to consider differential diagnoses) might overlook other morbidities. Ferris et al. (2002) explain that the frequency and severity of misdiagnosis of vaginal yeast infections are significant concerns. Inaccurate diagnosis can lead to delays in the treatment of more serious disorders. The example of yeast infection provides a useful heuristic, as we shall see. First, medical views are clearly divided as to whether this is a suitable condition for self-diagnosis. Second, it is a common condition. And third, the doctor no longer needs to serve as gatekeeper to treatment in many countries, because antifungal medication for its treatment is readily available without prescription.

The first approval for an over-the-counter (OTC) antifungal was made in the United States in 1990. Many other countries followed suit. This approval led to a reduction in prescription costs and physician services (Gurwitz, McLaughlin, and Fish 1995) but an increase in pharmaceutical sales (Ferris, Dekle, and Litaker 1996). The result of the switch from prescription to OTC medication was likely to have contributed to a shift of financial burden from the insurer to the health consumer (Harrington and Shepherd 2002).

Accompanying the switch to OTC status is the concomitant drive by the pharmaceutical industry to increase lay awareness of the condition, particularly in countries such as the United States and New Zealand where direct-to-consumer advertising (DTCA) is legal. Self-screening tools are prevalent in this drive for disease recognition, and they frequently appeal to emotional rather than clinical imperatives. The Monistat Web page provides an excellent example (Monistat 2009): "Try not to get too anxious. We'll help you figure out what's happening, why you are feeling the way you are, and most importantly, guide you in the right direction for a treatment that's right for you." It provides symptom lists and a "treatment finder" as well as lists of "questions for your doctor." A nurse practitioner is also available to answer questions submitted by women to the Web site. Research on DTCA indicates that, even when a woman ends up consulting her own doctor, advertising leads to more prescriptions for the advertised medicines regardless of what the doctor thinks about the treatment (Mintzes et al. 2002).

Self-diagnosis is not driven by the pharmaceutical industry alone. Online communities—some funded by the industry, others not—also promote disease awareness. The CFIDS (chronic fatigue and immune dysfunction syndrome) Association of America Web page, for example, provides an interactive screening tool to assess the probability of an individual having chronic fatigue syndrome (CFS), albeit with the caution "Only a doctor or qualified health professional can diagnose CFS. This assessment, however, can help you determine whether your symptoms may indicate CFS" (CFIDS Association of America 2009).

The contestable nature of such diseases as CFS helps to explain medical ambivalence, if not resentment, of lay prediagnosis (more on this in chapter 4). Until medicine officially sanctions particular conditions with a diagnostic label, it is reluctant to condone lay-driven disease campaigns (see P. Brown 1995).

On the other hand, self-diagnosis appears to be welcome in certain well-defined circumstances. Already, the emphasis on self-care and "concordance" (rather than compliance) seeks to cast the lay person as a decision maker (Mullen 1997). Extending the autonomy of the individual beyond care to diagnosis, however, is more unusual. Outside of the discussion of vaginal yeast infection, self-diagnosis has its most robust supporters in those conditions for which medical assistance is not available, is unreliable, or is a burden to the public health system.

The extreme examples of malaria and altitude sickness are conditions that tend to surface in geographic locations where doctors are rarely found. Self-diagnosis becomes an imperative, or at least an aspiration. But the closer-to-home example of H1N1 influenza virus is perhaps a more pertinent one. While the 2009–10 pandemic is too recent to feature as a subject of the sociological literature, the diagnosis of individual cases by lay people is a prominent feature of exposure control in public health literature. As mentioned above, self-diagnosis is a cornerstone of pandemic management. It falls under the category of "elimination of potential exposures," which is on the top level in the hierarchy of actions designed to minimize transmission of influenza (Centers for Disease Control and Prevention 2009). By minimizing outpatient visits for those with mild influenza-like illness, the self-diagnosed becomes self-isolated, concurrently reducing his or her opportunities to transmit the virus.

While this makes self-diagnosis of influenza highly desirable, there have been no studies to confirm its efficacy. The demedicalization of mild influenza presumes that individuals can distinguish among colds, influenza, pneumonia (or other lower respiratory infections), and other systemic illnesses. This may be correct, but it is untested. Researchers recently reported delays in treatment for potentially life-threatening illnesses that resulted from the incorrect diagnosis of influenza (Houlihan et al. 2010). Further, along with self-diagnosis comes self-treatment, and in many cases the rush toward oseltamivir (Tamiflu), which has been released in many countries as an OTC medication, creates the same commercial forces and potential conflicts as described above.

What makes this case interesting is that medicine has deemed that self-diagnosis is acceptable in this instance yet vigorously refutes its utility in lay-led, contested conditions where the consequences of misdiagnosis are arguably no more severe (see, for example, P. Brown 1995). This selective acceptance of self-diagnosis confirms the authoritative role of medicine, even while it enables individuals to decide for themselves what ails them. With respect to influenza infection, medicine remains the custodian of the diagnosis but determines who its delegates should be. Further, self-diagnosis presents challenges to the compliant "patient." While contemporary "consumers" may participate in their health care in new and autonomous ways, authorized self-diagnosis is nonetheless transformative and complex. As Henwood and colleagues' (2003) research shows, many individuals do not wish to assume responsibility for medical information and decision making. They indicate that it is the doctor's "job" and that ignorance about such matters is a relief rather than a source of disempowerment. Further, the skills required to seek, source, and appraise information are not within the ability, or even the interest, of all people. Finally, the nature of the doctor-patient relationship may not enable the enactment of an informed patient identity, particularly when the two are at odds.

There are no clear binaries to guide the incorporation of self-diagnosis into contemporary health management. It is a complex matter because it is a relational one, tightly bound up in the ways in which lay people and doctors position themselves and interact with one another.

What Next?

"What is the place of the patient in the co-production of a diagnosis?" asks Blaxter (2009). In the presence of new technologies, must the patient vanish? Similarly, we should perhaps ask, "Where does the doctor go in this new era of the patient consumer-expert-advocate?"

New models for the doctor-patient relationship abound. They focus on partnerships (Williamson 1999), concordance (Mullen 1997), coprovision (Buetow 2005), interpretation (Leder 1990), negotiation, productive alliance (Filc 2006), and homologization (Buetow, Jutel, and Hoare 2009). The patient may be involved, expert, compliant, autonomous, or resourceful. But the majority of these models focus on transformation of the patient identity *within* the dominant biomedical model. Medicine is still the final authority, enabling patient participation, albeit on a short lead. The "expert patients" manage their own care: monitoring symptoms, using the appropriate treatment, knowing how to optimize their well-being, and generally managing their illness independently from the doctor (Wilson 2001). This patient expertise implies compliance with the medical model, including acceptance of medicine's definition of disease. Yet, as Julia Neuberger has noted, "active" and "patient" are contradictory terms (Neuberger 1999; Wilson 2001, p. 135).

In spite of these changing dynamics, lay and expert knowledges retain their respective positions in the traditional hierarchy and give medicine the last word. This inequitable balance can explain the contested diagnoses that are discussed in the next chapter. It also explains why the integration of new players previously external to the doctor-patient relationship (such as technology and pharmaceutical firms, direct-to-consumer advertising, disease advocacy groups, managed care, and others) is experienced variably as introducing vulnerability and empowerment by doctors and patients alike. Nick Fox and Katie Ward's (2006) work on health identities is useful for understanding what is engendered by the changing status of patient and doctor in the diagnostic encounter: a paradox of both empowerment and disempowerment. Their empirical work reveals the blurring of identities in the independent patient. These may range from compliant to out-and-out rebellious, with the audacious "consumer" positioned somewhere in between. As health information flows across the Internet, some consume it as an adjunct to medical care, seeking online communities to be more assiduous or more expert in, say, the use of weight-loss medication. Discussing the ethnography of a weight-loss discussion list, Fox and Ward identify a group that sought to conform to biomedical expectations, incorporating medical opinion, specifically the opinion of users' individual GPs, to frame their activities. At the opposite extreme, women who have serious eating disorders used an online forum not to adhere to but rather to resist conventional medical treatment. The aim of that group was not to cure anorexia nervosa but to support individuals so diagnosed in circumventing the recommended medical approach.

Health identities, according to Fox and Ward, "are not prior, nor are they determined. Rather they emerge from concrete embodiment practices in relation to material, cultural, technological and emotional contexts" (N. Fox and Ward 2006, p. 475). Neither are the technologies of diagnosis or the diagnoses themselves prior and independent. Fox and Ward's model, which is based on Gilles Deleuze and Felix Guattari's ontology, demonstrates the confluence of factors that creates the identity of the individual. It comprises an assemblage that cannot overlook the diagnosis. The identities of both doctor and patient are defined not only by each another but by the pivotal diagnosis that sits between both as explanation, expectation, trophy, stigmata, assault, confounder, justification, key, identifier, and so on.

Returning to the chapter epigraph, consider Raymond Carver's interaction with his doctor. Imagine the situation were the diagnosis other than catastrophic malignancy. There would still be a relational element in what the diagnosis means and how it is incorporated into the patient's experience of health and illness. "The x-ray is clear. There's nothing wrong." (*Are you sure? Am I imagining this? Is it in my head? Do you know what you are doing?*) "It's just a bit of airway irritation. Should clear up when the pollen levels drop." (*Damned trees! Maybe I'll go have a weekend on the coast. Thanks for the news. You been to the coast recently? Where'd you go?*) "You need to stretch yourself more. You're out of breath because you're getting unfit." (*Should be more disciplined. Should go to the gym. Used to go jogging— when did I get so lazy? How 'bout your waist line? Don't act so damned superior!*)

Diagnosis brings lay person and professional together in a curiously intimate and consequential way, with the goal of achieving a better understanding of a problematic state of being. The ideal encounter is explanatory, predictive, and curative. However, as illustrated in the pages to come, diagnosis can be both a disputed object and an integral component of health identity. In a contested diagnosis, there is both an individual and a collective disappointment, which chapter 4 explores.

CHAPTER FOUR

Beyond Our Ken?

Contested Diagnoses and the Medically Unexplained

What happens when the chronically vulnerable person feels compelled to
be a patient? The homeostasis of the chronic vulnerable state dissolves in a
hunt for an elusive disease, a "monster that can be locked up with diagnosis." Months and even years pass, and no test result is sufficiently reproducible or specific to overwhelming uncertainty. The tragic patient is
drowning in Bayesian false starts. Faced with escalating illness, so discordant from demonstrable disease, medicine is not likely to accept blame
for subjecting the patient to months of an exercise that turned out to be
flawed in design and iatrogenic in execution. One option is to suggest
counseling of some ilk; more often than not, the patient hears, "You think
it's in my mind," and bridles at the affront to their perspicacity, if not
veracity. The battle is less likely to be joined if a diagnostic paralogism is
offered; these are labels that subsume pathogenetic hypotheses. They
promulgate a more vulnerable state by promising naught but palliation
until an answer is forthcoming from science—sometime in the future.

NORTIN M. HADLER, MD (1996)

W hen Phil Brown first called for a sociology of diagnosis in his 1995
paper "Naming and Framing," he used contested illness as the fulcrum
of his argument. He claimed that it is precisely because lay and professional
understandings of health and illness are different that the question of diagnosis is so important. The ways in which people experience illness do not
necessarily align with the ways medical knowledge classifies disease: "Diagnostic discovery is frequently laden with dispute, which provides a lens for
viewing many of the social conflicts which revolve around issues of medicine
and health" (P. Brown 1995, p. 38).

I discuss above how medical authority may transform the patient narrative, rendering foreign what was once personal. This is most salient in the
case of the contested diagnosis. A number of conditions—some common,
others idiosyncratic—find their recognition thwarted by medicine. They are

accepted neither by doctors nor by government or insurance companies yet are fully experienced by the individual as illness. This uncomfortable clash of perception is at the base of what is referred to as contested, or disputed, diseases. These are conditions that medicine does not acknowledge but the laity—be it an individual or a group of individuals who have what they believe to be the same condition—believe to be diseases. Sufferers often experience the defense of their illness as a battle, such as the one described by Dr. Hadler in the chapter epigraph. His words punctuate the degree to which contest or dispute is always potentially present in the diagnostic process, particularly in the case of the disability determination of someone who has a disputed diagnosis. The link to disability determination helps to explain dispute. It is, in turn, linked with resource allocation, transforming the doctor into gate-keeper (rather than explainer), with diagnosis as a key.

In the pages that follow, I look at a few of the ways in which disease designation results in social conflict, likely to push the individual to contest a diagnosis or its absence. I then use the example of the medically unexplained symptom to demonstrate the discursive construction of illness that medicine cannot (or will not) currently label. Finally, I consider ways in which the contest in lay-professional interactions may be receding, or at least changing. Here, my focus is mainly on collective discord. Where do lay and professional beliefs collide over what counts as a disease and what responses does either party assume in the case of contest?

Dumit (2006) defines five characteristics that link contested diagnoses. First, these diseases are frequently chronic. They do not fit the acute disease model and, consequently, do not enable simple cost calculations. Second, they have uncertain etiology and are frequently "biomental," meaning their cause is attributed variably to physical, social, toxic exposure, or psychiatric causes. Third, their treatment is diverse and may be approached by various therapeutic avenues, including alternative medicine. Fourth, their boundaries are unclear and they have many comorbidities. While professionals might argue that they are psychogenic, patients might retort that their obvious depression is the result of the disregard in which they are held by the medical fraternity. Finally, they are "legally explosive," notably as a result of their link to disability assignment. If the conditions are not recognized as disease, people who have them are not entitled to compensation for treatment or for the changes the illnesses impose on their lifestyles.

Numerous conditions fit this bill. Fibromyalgia is one such ailment. It is a contested diagnosis of exclusion that may be proposed when a panoply of other potential medical explanations fail to explain chronic widespread pain, sleep disturbance, fatigue, and bilateral tender points. The etiology is uncertain, and indeed it is often referred to as psychogenic in nature. There is no therapeutic agreement as to how fibromyalgia should be managed, and the diagnosis is clearly linked to disability allocation (Sim and Madden 2008).

The pursuit of diagnosis emerges as one of the most pressing issues identified by people who have the condition. The symptoms they experienced are so incapacitating that they feel they must have undetected malignancy but have been told by doctors that nothing is wrong and that their symptoms are psychological in nature, despite the distinctly physical manner in which they experience these symptoms themselves. They speak of resentment for what they perceive to be a dismissive approach to their suffering. With fibromyalgia, receiving a diagnosis is initially a relief because it validates their illness, reassures them about the absence of malignancy, and gives them a sense of credibility, lost in the prediagnosis process. However, the diagnosis of fibromyalgia is not uniformly welcomed either. People who have it feel they need to keep the diagnosis secret to avoid stigmatization. Some feel health care professionals believe their fibromyalgia is not legitimate and are quickly disinterested in the patients if cure is not prompt (Sim and Madden 2008).

Closely related to fibromyalgia is chronic fatigue syndrome. Like fibromyalgia, it includes the conditions Dumit enumerates as requisite for a contested diagnosis. CFS is a chronic, disabling physical and mental fatigue of uncertain etiology and with no agreed-upon treatment (Deale and Wessely 2001). This syndrome, which those who have it find completely incapacitating, is often met with dismissal and disbelief by doctors. Deale and Wessely found that two-thirds of patients who had CFS were dissatisfied with medical care and received what they believed was an inappropriate psychiatric diagnosis. Patients believe strongly that the symptoms are indicative of physical illness, while many doctors believe in the psychological origin of the disease (Deale and Wessely 2001).

Contest is accentuated by the latent dichotomy between illness and disease, the unequal power relationship between patient and doctor, and the need for a medical diagnosis before other services can be accessed. Contest, notably in emerging illnesses such as Hadler's example of fibromyalgia, assumes a particularly acute form when the absence of diagnosis denies the patient access to the sick role and (more important) to institutional recognition of suffering.

Many have written of the distress of patients who do not receive a diagnosis for their complaint. This distress typically focuses on disorder, confusion, and fear of service denial or of being stigmatized by a psychogenic explanation (Dumit 2006; Nettleton 2006; Malterud 2001, 2005).

Dumit (2006) describes how conflict is shaped both within and outside of the patient-doctor relationship. Clinicians are directed in their practice by the impositions of the health maintenance organization, the employer, and the insurer; bureaucracy determines who can provide care and for which ailments. These organizations, combined, have symbolic domination over the individual patient. But the key point, as Dumit makes clear, is "the intense interplay between diagnosis and legitimacy: without a diagnosis and other forms of acceptance into the medical system, sufferers are at risk of being denied social recognition of their very suffering and accused of simply faking it" (p. 578).

Contested diagnoses are typically those that cannot currently be explained by medicine or that have explanations that are in dispute (P. Brown and Zavestoski 2004). The contest focuses on debate around whether they are primarily social, psychiatric, or biological in nature (Dumit 2006). These are illnesses that are "are not defined in terms of organic pathology, but on the basis of their symptoms" (Nettleton et al. 2004). I discuss in the paragraphs that follow how the medical literature deals with medically unexplained, enigmatic symptoms. The difficulty of living with the uncertainty of nondiagnosis and of defending the legitimacy of complaints results in significant distress and dissatisfaction with the medical profession (Nettleton 2006).

Conversely, conflict may also arise when diagnosis achieves nonclinical ends and therefore stymies the rights of the patient, who does not believe him- or herself to be ill. A powerful example is political psychiatry, where dissent is treated as mental illness. Robin Munro (2002) quotes a Chinese textbook that develops the notion of "political mania" as a form of paranoid psychosis: "Those afflicted do avid research into politics and put forward a whole set of original theories of their own, which they then try to peddle by every means possible. . . . [S]uch people are sometimes viewed as being political dissidents" (Sifa Jingshen Yixue Jianding Zixun Jieda, qtd. in Munro 2002). During the Cultural Revolution in China, the Revolutionary Committee provided oversight of psychiatry and its diagnostic practices, requiring political justification of diagnostic and treatment decision making for mental health patients (Yip 2005).

Similar political control of diagnostic categories figures in Russian psychiatry. Coercive psychiatry was widely used well into the 1980s to hospitalize political and religious dissidents in the absence of psychiatric illness. What enabled this detention were laws that allowed medical custody of individuals who had committed a crime but were "nonimputable" because of mental illness. Antipsychotic medication was used in high doses to treat "delusions of reformism" and "anti-Soviet thoughts" (Bonnie 2002, pp. 137–38).

Lest readers assume that the politicization of diagnosis is restricted to repressive regimes, the more conventional diagnoses of antisocial personality disorder and dangerous and severe personality disorder (DSPD) bear mentioning. As Corbett and Westwood (2005) point out, many of the diagnostic criteria for antisocial personality disorder identified in the DSM-IV may be typical within particular subcultures and actually emerge as a result of alienation by or from dominant norms and values (e.g., failure to conform to social norms, deceitfulness, failure to plan ahead, irritability or aggressiveness, disregard for safety, failure to sustain consistent work or pay debts, lack of remorse regarding hurting or stealing from another, and the individual's being at least 18 years of age) (pp. 124–25).

DSPD is a diagnosis that, Corbett and Westwood (2005) argue, emerges from a risk-averse society anxious to provide a perception of safety in the context of a highly sensationalized debate about the relationship between psychiatric diseases and violence. In this case, the idea that individuals may present risk to social order above and beyond the preexisting health laws is embodied in the diagnosis.

Medically Unexplained Symptoms

The issue of the nondiagnosable medical complaint takes a curious role, challenging medicine's modus operandi, which seeks to identify and treat disease. Where medicine is not able to label a patient's affliction within its available diagnostic frameworks, its discursive approach reveals much about how medicine considers conditions that are baffling or not easily classified.

The phrase "medically unexplained symptoms" would seem self-explanatory. There are physical symptoms that bring patients to consult but for which doctors cannot establish a cause. The discursive approach of both medical literature and practice is paradoxical—transforming the range of unexplained causes for consultation into a unitary condition with its own diagnostic label, linking it to psychiatric dysfunction, augmenting patient suffering, and failing to appraise critically the limitations of its episteme. In the following pages, I make that critical appraisal by reviewing the role of the symptom, appraising the current literature that focuses on the medically unexplained symptom, and identifying how medical discourses about medically explained symptoms shift responsibility for illness to the patient and interfere with the interpretative role of the doctor.

The Symptom

Foucault (1963) described how the symptom took on a new role in nineteenth-century clinical medicine. Previously the sole locus of medical interest, it became instead a key, a clue, or a pointer to deeper and more significant conditions. This is what the taxonomists and the nosologists had been attempting to clarify as they assembled symptoms into diagnostic classifications. The arrangement of these symptoms were a window to otherwise hidden disease. "Cough, chest pain, and shortness of breath are not pleurisy. . . . They are its essential symptoms," wrote Foucault (p. 89, my translation). No longer were symptoms considered as individual phenomena; they became the external expression of disease. This transformed the doctor's role into one of detective: unscrambling the messages of the symptom to discover the link between signifier and pathology.

Drew Leder (1990) describes this stealth work as an interpretive process. The patient brings to the medical consultation a situation that he or she is not fully able to interpret but has assigned to the medical realm. In the desire to understand the discomfort, the cough, the rash, the swelling, or the cramp, the patient initiates an encounter with the doctor. This is what the doctor will refer to as the symptom: a "subjective" experience or change in function. In turn, the doctor channels the narrative of illness or dysfunction toward an interpretive outcome, asking questions about personal and family history, querying both the presentation and absence of symptoms. The doctor then undertakes a physical assessment, exploring the body-object—now silent while palpated, auscultated, and measured—to create a narrative that explains the patient's complaint. Finally, both patient and doctor acquiesce to the numerical findings contained in instrumental texts such as x-ray, scans, blood count, or manometer.

This encounter is guided by a presumptive paradigm and measured by clinical efficacy. This means that prediagnosis conceptions underpin the manner in which the doctor explores the complaint and prevent an aimless "fishing trip" of nonsystematic explorations and questions. The collection of symptoms, along with the patient's story, points the doctor in a particular direction, suggesting a collection of potential diagnoses or explanations and reducing the complexity of decision making (Croskerry 2002). It also means that the encounter cannot be considered successful if medical interpretation emerging from the interaction does not result in the patient's cooperative comprehension or in clinical improvement.

Yet anywhere from 10 to 35 percent of primary consultations fail to alleviate the presenting complaint. Frustrated by symptoms for which they cannot find a recognized medical diagnosis, doctors devote much energy to explaining and identifying a presumed root cause. This entails a significant financial and structural impact on health care, generates inappropriate referrals and treatment, frustrates physicians, and of course, results in distress for the patient, who generally consults with the hope of identifying an explanation and concordant cure.

The term "medically unexplained symptom" and its impact is the subject of increasing reflection in the medical literature. A critical review of articles focusing on these enigmatic symptoms demonstrates a growing concern with the burdens they present for patients, doctors, and the health care system but also reveals a curious approach to the problem.[1] Paradoxically, many of the articles resort to creating a catchall diagnostic category in which it can place the unexplained.[2] The phrase "medically unexplained symptoms" is frequently used interchangeably with psychiatric diagnostic terms such as somatoform disorder, somatizing, functional somatic syndrome, and other related terms implying a condition of psychogenic or sociogenic origin. The place of the medically unexplained symptom is an important diagnostic component of these conditions, but in these articles medically unexplained symptoms are subsumed within the psychiatric disorders and used synonymously. On the other hand, a modest proportion of these articles critique the tendency to provide a psychogenic explanation, to diagnose by exclusion, or to recognize the limitations of medical knowledge vis-à-vis the physical complaints of patients. I discuss this at greater length below.

But whether the publications see medically unexplained symptoms as psychogenic or not, there is a pervasive reference to them as an entity, or as a unified condition that could be considered under one light. The literature links medically unexplained symptoms semantically with phrases such as "the *prob-*

lem of medically unexplained symptoms," "*diagnosing* medically unexplained symptoms," and "*treating* medically unexplained symptoms." This semantic formulation reduces chronic fatigue, lower back pain, irritable bowel syndrome, and so on to the unitary label of medically unexplained symptoms. The use of the acronym "MUS" reifies the notion that all physical complaints without explanation can be viewed in the same way. But it is not just nomenclature. References to medically unexplained symptoms as a *diagnosis*, a *problem* to be approached epidemiologically, or a treatable or preventable *condition* and to those who have them as a homogenous group confirm that this is an approach that reasons through diagnosis rather than interpretation.

Psychiatry to Explain the Unexplainable

Rosenberg (2006) writes that "psychiatry is the residuary legatee of . . . developments that have always been contested at the ever-shifting boundary between disease and deviance, feeling and symptom, the random and the determined, the stigmatized and the value-free" (p. 237). He seeks here to account for how disease categories explain behavior and emotional pain. This is relevant to the issue of medically unexplained symptoms, as the seemingly unjustified symptoms are "behaviors" in a model that uses psychiatry to explain the unexplained. This psychiatric domiciliation of the unexplained is problematic because it frequently relies on diagnosis by exclusion (settled on by ruling out other explanations), fails to acknowledge the limitations of knowledge, and shifts responsibility for cause and cure in a way that ignores sociohistorical realities.

First, considering medically unexplained symptoms a psychiatric disorder is a diagnosis by exclusion. In other words, it is a diagnosis made not on the basis of what it is but on the basis of what it is not. The absence of explanation, rather than the presence of a well-defined feature, defines the condition. The label becomes a wastebasket diagnosis—a classification in which may be placed many conditions that don't easily fit elsewhere. As Robins and Helzer (1986) point out, psychiatric diagnosis is already challenged by the absence of definitive tests to mark the presence of a disorder; there is no equivalent to the x-ray of orthopedics or the hemoculture of infectious disease. It is therefore difficult to establish a positive diagnosis yet facile to attach a positive psychiatric diagnosis to a medical patient.

Second, this assumption of psychiatric disorder in the absence of other diagnoses presumes the infallibility of the doctor and of the field. And yet one postmortem study revealed errors of diagnosis in 39 percent of major diagnoses and 50 percent of less serious diagnoses (Aalton, Samson, and Jansen 2006). Numerous diagnostic errors can be retrospectively assigned to an incomplete knowledge of the field. For example, Lyme disease, before its designation as a specific diagnosable entity, was often cast as atypical rheumatoid arthritis (Graber, Gordon, and Franklin 2002); multiple sclerosis was frequently diagnosed as a psychiatric disorder, possibly because of the subjective nature of many early symptoms (Skegg, Corwin, and Skegg 1988). Symptoms may also be atypical, presenting challenges for clinician and patient alike (Malterud and Taksdal 2007).

Advances in genetic understandings of illness provide links between pathologies that were previously seen as completely distinct (F. Miller et al. 2006). As Kirmayer et al. (2004) state, "The lack of explanation reflects the limits of medical knowledge, available technology and the epistemological difficulties of assigning a clear cause to subjective complaints like pain and fatigue, which may have no objectively measurable correlates and may change rapidly over time in quality and intensity" (p. 663).

Third, this approach to the unexplained symptom shifts responsibility (for the inability to explain the symptom) from the doctor to the patient, positing the cause as the patient's mental health. Hadler (1996) reflects on both causes and limitations of this blanket psychogenic labeling, describing medicine as "not likely to accept blame for subjecting the patient to months of an exercise that turn[s] out to be flawed in design and iatrogenic in execution." Similarly, Nettleton (2006) reports that the effort to palliate symptoms in the absence of a diagnosis is as onerous as the symptoms themselves. "Society does not readily give people permission to be ill," she writes, "in the absence of an 'accepted' abnormal pathology or physiology" (p. 1176).

Pilowsky (1994) claims that the contest of diagnosis is weighted toward the physician. He defines abnormal illness behavior as an "inappropriate or maladaptive mode of experiencing . . . one's own state of health which persists despite the fact that an appropriate social agent . . . has an accurate and reasonably lucid explanation of the nature of the person's health status." He does point out that the doctor's potential to err is an important liability of this definition and that in some cases there is a hasty progression from lack of explanation to considering a patient's behavior "abnormal." Salient in Pilowsky's definition is the recognition of the important yet equivocal role of the "social agent" or doctor.

Locating the symptom in psychology ascribes responsibility and moral blame in a way that encourages patient resistance (Kirmayer et al. 2004). While a physical explanation for a symptom confers, in most cases, a lack of personal responsibility for its onset, a psychiatric one implies that the patient might have the ability to both control and reverse the physical symptoms, an interpretation that may seem impossible to the patient and that brings with it stigma and shame.

Finally, a psychogenic explanation relies for diagnostic criteria on histori-cally and socially developed patterns of behavior that emerge from the ex-pectations of modern medicine. An important criterion in the "diagnosis" of "MUS" is frequency of GP attendance. Against the background I have in-troduced above, repeated consultations for complaints that have no readily visible disease explanation may be the result of compliance with social expec-tations about the role of the doctor and of medicine.

For example, a mother is rewarded for the medicalization of her children's health. Many countries provide financial or other incentives for parents to engage in "well-child" checkups. Direct-to-consumer advertising admonishes the public, "Check with your doctor and find out if X is right for you!" using enticing and effective models to elicit consumption of specific pharmaceutical products and medical care generally. General medical practice may include such nonmedical services as family planning and ear piercing. Women are far greater consumers of these services than men and are more often sub-ject to, and compliant with, calls to consult the doctor, resulting in a greater prevalence of "diagnosed" MUS. This compliance is historically learned from the medicalization of women's health, as featured in (but not restricted to) the menstrual disability theory. Based on the Newtonian concept that en-ergy can neither be created nor destroyed, this approach to women's health, originating in the nineteenth century, held that the periodic bleeding of the woman represented the loss of vital energy (Vertinsky 1994). Because women are "eternally injured," they are transformed into docile subjects who sought medical attention readily. Subsequently, they become unequally slotted into the category of psychiatric illness by exclusion. Malterud's work submits that clinical approach is based on gender and detrimentally traps women into diagnostic categories and treatment protocols (Malterud 1999, 2000, 2001; Malterud, Candid, and Code 2004).

Health promotion organizations, on the other hand, lament the noncom-pliance of men, who are less likely than women to see their doctor regularly. A growing body of literature points out that men have poor help-seeking behavior, are reluctant to consult a GP until well past the propitious time (Galdas, Cheater, and Marshall 2005), and are more reliant on social factors than on the gravity of symptoms to determine when they will consult (Wolters et al. 2002). Poor help-seeking behavior on the part of men is proposed as one of the reasons for worse health outcomes in men than in women (Galdas, Cheater, and Marshall 2005). Addressing this deficiency is an important focus of men's health initiatives (McKinlay 2005). Because men are often reluctant to consult a GP, alternatives have been developed, including using sports clubs and pubs as venues for health promotion activities.

How, Then, to Explain the Unexplained?

I have shown the limitations of "diagnosing" medically unexplained symptoms as an entity. It is a diagnosis of exclusion, which presumes the infallibility of the physician and the omniscience of medicine. It transfers responsibility for the disorder to the patient, and it ignores sociohistorical practices that influence patient behavior and place women unequally under scrutiny for psychogenic disorder.

There is, however, a range of ways of explaining complaints that are not linked with disease. Returning to Leder's hermeneutic contextualization of the patient-doctor encounter, we can easily see that one explanation is that the patient has incorrectly attributed the origin of her complaint to the realm of medicine. While the experiential text may not legitimately have its explanation in medicine, medicine's role as arbitrator may lead the patient to presume the contrary. And industry marketing's use of the stamp of medical approval to sell its wares enhances the chances of the patient's making assumptions about the medical nature of the complaints (P. Conrad and Leiter 2004).

Many serious symptoms and dysfunctions affecting digestion, mobility, comfort, and kinesthesia may be quite clearly "real" without being medical. The tortuous course of lower back pain in the absence of structural pathology may be explained by a muscle-balance assessment, and "cured" by development of core strength and exercise prescription rather than by surgical, medical, or pharmacological solutions (Abenhaim et al. 2000). Similarly, bloating, flatulence, diarrhea, and other digestive system distress that cannot be explained by celiac disease or some other defined clinical entity may still be related to dietary intolerances and obscure food allergies that a nutritionist could better address (see, for example, Meador's [2005] unusual case study of a specific brand of toothpaste as a causative factor in intractable diarrhea). A biomechanical explanation may be at the heart of a number of functional disorders that an occupational therapist, clinical biomechanist, or podiatrist would be better suited than either physician or surgeon to diagnose and correct.

In the same way, unknown and unexpected environmental factors may explain any number of respiratory, gastroenteric, cutaneous, and functional symptoms. Many conditions that are medically unexplained overlap strongly with explained conditions, such as asthma. Environmental factors are an underresearched area of potential explanation and are often contested diagnoses, reflecting sociopolitical forms of illness in the case of unacknowledged environmental contamination, for example (P. Brown 1995; Kipen and Fiedler 2002).

A condition may be medical but not recognized as such. Inclusion in the ICD is by application. To be considered, a condition must first be recognized and then championed. Some conditions are functional and treatable but are not linked to a particular pathology. Radiotherapy damage, whiplash sequelae, and even the common cough (A. Goldstein 2007) can be discrete entities of their own that we could perhaps understand as physical dysfunctions rather than as diseases.

Finally, we need to consider that the explanation *may* be psychiatric. Physical symptoms are recognized as part of psychiatric syndromes. They are a common comorbidity in major depressive disorder (Arnow et al. 2006), are part of the diagnostic criteria for generalized anxiety (American Psychiatric Association 2000), are often linked with psychosis, and so on. Psychiatry is a legitimate form of medicine and has a diagnostic framework for disease, as does physical medicine. However, psychogenic disease should not be a diagnosis by exclusion. It should be determined based on positive findings in the context of a comprehensive biopsychosocial assessment.

Discovery of Disease

I have discussed the fact that classification is a human endeavor that involves parceling a continuum of nature into discrete packages that make sense to those who are in the business of differentiating the particular conditions at hand. How, then, does a disease come to be classified? The way in which a particular set of symptoms become accepted as one thing and not another must be part of how we understand diagnosis and its impact. This is what Phil Brown (1995) refers to as the "disease discovery process."

Brown proposes a model for disease discovery. Unlike other models (for example, Peter Conrad and Joseph Schneider's [1980] model of medicalization), Brown's provides a mechanism for understanding the roles that lay people and the medical institution play in the establishment of diagnoses, including those where lay and professional views might not agree. His model identifies distinct factors that are typically part of the disease discovery process but are not present in all disease discovery and are not sequential. They do, in any case, demonstrate how consensus, politics, and interest must converge before a diagnostic category can exist. There are four elements in Brown's model: lay discovery, social movement, professional factors, and institutional and organizational factors.

Whether a disease is contested or not will depend on the degree to which lay people and medicine agree on the nature of a particular condition. This agreement in turn is likely to be influenced by a range of factors, as described by Dumit and discussed above in this chapter. How unusual is the symptomatology? What are the treatment regimens? Can the condition be cast as psychogenic? Are there resources at stake?

The histories of individual diseases illustrate how these factors interact to generate diagnoses.[3] Wilbur Scott's account of the incorporation of post-traumatic stress disorder (PTSD) into the DSM-III provides a detailed account of the considerable individual and collective effort required to obtain acknowledgement that the psychological distress of numerous Vietnam veterans was something different from the psychosis, cowardice, or malingering to which it had previously been attributed (W. Scott 1990). The effort was political, involving negotiation, relationship management, and persuasion. Scott recounts this as an example of how diagnosis brings conditions forward as "always-already-there objects in the world" (p. 295) via a convincing display of objective evidence: "a discovery of what was present but previously unseen" (p. 295). The agents in this particular political process were cognizant of the fact that it did not suffice for the condition to be, as they saw it, a real-thing-in-the-world; those with control over classificatory processes needed to be made to face the realness of the diagnosis. This could be accomplished only by concerted and repeated efforts. Choosing how to speak of the disorder, with whom to discuss it, when to have discussions, and how to use collective action were instrumental factors in the campaign to have PTSD included in the DSM-III.

Wilbur Scott's (1990) description brings to the fore each step in Phil Brown's (1995) model of social discovery. Lay discoveries by individual veterans, buttressed by the social movement of veteran organizations, were pivotal in the acceptance of PTSD in the DSM-III. Before its introduction as a diagnosis, there was an acknowledged interest in the psychiatric casualties of combat. These had been observed to be both immediate and delayed. However, in the Vietnam era, despite the frequent clinical observation and reports of deeply stressed veterans, there was no classification in the DSM that met the description of their distress or that encouraged the inclusion of a description of the war experience as part of the diagnostic pathway.

The development of a postcombat stress disorder was to emerge from a combination of lay and professional forces committed to the welfare of returning military personnel. As Brown notes is to be expected in lay-led discovery, the promotion of this particular label required professional backing of the lay movement. Robert Lifton and Chaim Shaton, both psychiatrists with strong antiwar sentiments, joined the Vietnam Veterans against the War "rap sessions." These meetings had a political purpose of consolidating and disseminating information about the horrors of the war to the public but also provided an opportunity for a kind of street-corner psychiatry that enabled Lifton and Shaton to witness and gather information about a post-Vietnam syndrome (W. Scott 1990).

At almost the same time, the DSM-III revisions were being undertaken. News of the demedicalization of homosexuality opened the way for the introduction of many other changes to the diagnostic manual. Shaton, Lifton, and Sarah Haley, a social worker at the Boston Veterans Administration Hospital whose own family history of exposure to war atrocities made her particularly sensitive to the reports of her patients, joined with the director of the National Veterans Resource Project to launch a working group on postcombat disorder (W. Scott 1990). This lay-professional working group devoted itself to gathering empirical evidence of the disorder and to enlisting the political support of personalities in the psychiatric community (notably, Robert Spitzer, who was the director of the task force on nomenclature). Their work was successful, and in 1978, the Committee on Reactive Disorders of the American Psychiatric Association recommended the diagnostic label of "post-traumatic stress disorder" (W. Scott 1990).

Gulf War–related illnesses—like chronic fatigue syndrome, multiple chemical sensitivity, and fibromyalgia—serve as examples of medically unexplained symptoms and provide other examples of lay activism playing an important role in disease recognition. As many as 70,000 Gulf War veterans have sought treatment for illnesses that they believe are the result of exposure to environmental hazards during service (Zavestoski et al. 2002). They have reported such symptoms as nausea, loss of concentration, irritable bowels, and blurred vision. Two conflicting explanations are presented to explain these symptoms: on one hand, exposure to environmental hazards, such as anti–nerve gas pills, nerve agents such as sarin, pesticides, insect repellents, and the smoke from oil fires, tent heaters, and the burning of human waste; but on the other, traumatic psychological stress (Proctor et al. 1998).

The Department of Veteran Affairs (VA) initially denied care for such ailments on the basis that the symptoms were the result of stress, not of toxic exposure (Zavestoski et al. 2002). A National Institutes of Health technology workshop concluded that veteran illnesses were caused by PTSD, which manifested through nonspecific, multisystem physical symptoms rather than the flashbacks generally typical of the disorder (Zavestoski et al. 2002). Veterans resisted this label, partly because it did not necessarily guarantee access to services and treatment. Veterans also felt that such a conclusion was simply convenient for the Department of Defense, drawing attention away from its liability for the illnesses suffered by the veterans by minimizing the focus on environmental exposure. Veterans continued to push for more research into potential environmental hazards (Zavestoski et al. 2002). Gulf War veterans framed their inability to get the recognition and treatment they felt they were entitled to as an injustice, drawing on the experiences of Vietnam vets who were exposed to Agent Orange (P. Brown and Zavestoski 2004).

Veterans began to speak out, and increased media coverage resulted in collective mobilization. In 1994, the VA began providing care as a consequence of legislation requiring benefits for all chronically disabled veterans with undiagnosed disease. Yet many veterans still felt they were not getting the care they deserved (Zavestoski et al. 2002). Many felt betrayed by the government's refusal to provide them treatment and its insistence that there was not enough science to support their claims.

The veterans' actions are an example of health social movements (HSMs). These movements constitute a political force that address a number of problems as experienced by lay people and, in so doing, constitute a challenge to political power, professional authority, and personal and collective identity (P. Brown and Zavestoski 2004). The focus of HSMs may include access to care or to services, recognition of diseases, and inequality with regard to particular social groups. The way in which HSMs operate has been influenced by an era of scientization. Among other things, HSMs engage with medical science and public health to produce their own research and knowledge generation (P. Brown and Zavestoski 2004). The movements are thus attempting to democratize the production of knowledge in order to challenge traditional assumptions about causation and prevention, thus engaging more successfully in policy advocacy, research direction, and resource allocation (P. Brown and Zavestoski 2004).

One figuration of the health social movement is the "embodied health movement," which is organized so as to achieve medical recognition along with treatment and research for a particular illness or disease. Embodied health movements challenge science on etiology, diagnosis, treatment, and prevention by mobilizing medical professionals and scientists. Other examples of embodied health movements include the breast cancer, AIDS, and tobacco control movements (P. Brown and Zavestoski 2004). The experience of those with the disease plays an important role. AIDS activists, for example, managed to establish themselves as experts on the illness and were then able to have a significant influence on the production of knowledge, thus shaping policies and influencing research into treatments (Epstein 1996).

The exemplar embodied health movement is the environmental breast cancer movement. Breast cancer was constructed as a problem of insufficient knowledge, not a stigma or a problem of access to quality treatment. This linked breast cancer to institutional and governmental neglect and a failure to prioritize research funds. Activists successfully articulated their concerns to the general public and politicians through media coverage of the movement's activities (Kolker 2004). Breast cancer was subsequently constructed not as an individual problem but as a crisis for the general public. This was accomplished using three sets of culturally resonant frames in both the media and congressional hearings. First, breast cancer was framed as an epidemic; second, it was framed as a problem of gender equity; and third, it was framed as a threat to families (Kolker 2004).

In contrast, the discovery of Alzheimer disease was not lay initiated but owes its current position in public awareness to lay efforts. Alzheimer disease, which was named in the early twentieth century, was promoted by neurological researchers, and lay participation played a much later role, one that is notable more for the promotion of the diagnosis than for its creation. Scientific advancement, interprofessional relationships, and a particular cultural context enabled the discovery of this now renowned diagnosis.

Two different neuropathological schools (in Munich, where Alois Alzheimer worked in Emil Kraepelin's laboratory, and in Prague, where Oskar Fischer worked under Arnold Pick) were involved in a range of discoveries that were to frame Alzheimer disease (Amaducci, Rocca, and Schoenberg 1986). Previous medical literature described dementia in purely clinical terms and linked it with normal aging. The introduction of new staining and autopsy results enabled Alzheimer and his colleagues to identify "neurofibrillary tangles." Simultaneously, presumably using similar technology, Fischer described "senile plaques." Both lesions are considered characteristic of what we call Alzheimer disease today. However, scientific rivalry between the schools at Munich and Prague, and between Alzheimer and Fischer, resulted in a range of explanatory claims and descriptions for these disorders. These included Fischer plaques, Fischer presbyophenia, and, of course, the now-assimilated Alzheimer disease (Amaducci, Rocca, and Schoenberg 1986).

The nosological discussion was not resolved by technological advances but by Kraepelin, the director of the department in which Alzheimer worked. Kraepelin was a researcher whose own work was devoted to the classification of psychiatric disorders and disease categories. He assigned his junior's name to the diagnosis of presenile dementia. Amaducci and colleagues (1986) surmise that this action was taken to consolidate the position both of Kraepelin's school and of his researcher, and they comment that Kraepelin's reputation and authority were of primary importance in the creation and perpetuation of this particular diagnosis. It would probably also be safe to assume that Kraepelin's particular focus on taxonomy (see Kahn 1957) may have contributed to his interest and success in assigning the name to the condition.

Patrick Fox (1989) further maintains that the context of medicine at the time of these discoveries enabled the creation of this diagnosis. Alzheimer believed that the changes he saw in brain tissue were due to more than just aging. Fox writes: "The elimination of the age criterion was central because it contributed to the transformation of what had been generally considered 'senility' into a specific disease with specific pathological characteristics and symptoms" (p. 59). Fox also describes the push from family members of people who have Alzheimer disease, which, from the mid-twentieth century, rallied behind the Alzheimer disease label to bring it forward in public consciousness, generate research interest, and promote its diagnostic status as well as its characterization as a leading cause of death.

Many other diseases, on the other hand, remain in flux, perceived as medical diseases to lay patients but not accepted as such by medicine. These are in the throes of being variably discovered or discarded. As Phil Brown (1995) points out, the degree to which medicine might resist the incorporation of a condition as diagnosis depends on innumerable factors. Iatrogenicity, stigma, stereotypes, and corporate responsibility are all barriers to lay-led campaigns for disease recognition.

Whose Diagnosis?

Numerous pressures are chipping away at medicine's authority to diagnose. Whether this reduces or increases contest is to be seen. I discuss these in greater depth in other chapters, but I refer to some of them here for the purpose of exploring how these pressures contribute to a changing balance in the diagnostic contest.

First, there is a distinct change in the lay-professional relationship, as discussed in chapter 3. There have been changes in the roles that lay and medical practitioner play in their interactions, with what Buetow et al. (2009) refer to as homologization, or a role convergence, with reduced social distances between doctors and patient. The wider access to medical information has fueled this changing relationship, where mutually accessed information may converge, yet some differences persist and even widen, as evidenced by demand for particular remedies.

This is not to say that medicine no longer has authority. The biomedical expertise of those trained to practice medicine still carries much weight (Lupton 1997a). The practice of medicine, as well as its authority, is socially contingent and is framed by broader sociotechnological change (Nettleton 2004). Nettleton discusses this change and speaks of the informatization of medicine, where the body is seen as a system of information networks: the art of medicine gives way to evidence-based practice, the physical body defers to the CT scan, information once restricted to medicine is now available to the lay Web surfer, and the doctor-patient relationship becomes a meeting of experts.

Second, medicine's jurisdiction is shifting, incorporating new agents and social forces in its contemporary context. Among these are commercial agents, such as the pharmaceutical industry. Linked to this industry, and in the context of increased lay engagement with medical information, is the trend toward self-diagnosis.

Many pharmaceutical marketing Web sites provide a range of tools to encourage individuals to diagnose themselves and to present the diagnosis to the doctor and request the recommended treatment. The tools may include simple descriptions in lay language about features of a particular disease, checklists of risk factors, symptom diaries, and other online symptom assessment tests. This approach fits in neatly with the previously described increasing role of the patient in the doctor-patient encounter. Encouraging the patient to preidentify specific conditions before consulting the doctor is an important cornerstone of the disease branding strategies that seek to drive the market to recognize the presence of disease more widely and direct both patients and caregivers in the way they see particular pathologies (Parry 2007).

As discussed in chapter 3, self-diagnosis is not yet held in high regard by the medical profession and is considered useful only in certain circumstances. There seem to be two situations in which self-diagnosis is condoned by medicine. The first is when there is a public health imperative—that is to say, when population health is likely to be improved if lay people are able to diagnose either a contagious or a serious disease (and when early detection contributes to reduced morbidity). The second is with common benign disorders.

Where practitioners consistently draw the line in their tolerance of self-diagnosis is when it presents what Barsky and Borus (1999) refer to as "embattled advocacy," or self-diagnosis as a gesture of defiance to critique the judgment of the doctor. These authors describe a "self-perpetuating, self-validating cycle in which common, endemic, somatic symptoms are incorrectly attributed to serious abnormality, reinforcing the patient's belief that he or she has a serious disease" (p. 910).

Diagnosis offers a tool for political engagement in response to the rejection of disease claims. Diagnoses such as PTSD, black lung, and environmental disease offer a social view for victims of abuse or toxic exposure, opening the door to care and to compensation (P. Brown 1995). Diagnosis also provides a focus for a growing number of Internet communities. Web pages play a part in the social health movement, gathering individuals around existing and emerging diseases, both contested and accepted. These Internet communities offer an alternative support structure when the absence of diagnosis impugns the medical legitimacy of the individual's complaint (Dumit 2006). These communities "create their own separate and distinct medical culture, a culture that gives primary importance to the role of subjective experience" (D. Goldstein 2004, p. 127). Examples of virtual communities creating an alternative culture are the proanorexia sites that seek to redefine anorexia nervosa outside of medical discourse, casting it instead as a sanctuary, a "place where control and purity [can] be found" (N. Fox, Ward, and O'Rourke 2005, p. 958). Conversely, Internet communities are also launched by health providers who have identified Web pages as sites at which patients can be transformed from consumers into a "community of practice" with potentially improved health outcomes (Winkelman and Choo 2003).

In a general sense, virtual communities provide a sanctuary for alternative and stigmatized groups. Notable for their genesis in medical-lay discord about diagnosis, these groups may provide support for illnesses that medicine does not sanction. On the other hand, they may reject diagnostic classification, seeking to redefine what medicine perceives as disease in other terms (for example, see N. Fox, Ward, and O'Rourke's work on the proanorexia movement [2005] or St-Onge, Provencher, and Ouellet on psychosis [2005]). Or they may accept diagnosis and reject the curtailing of what are more generally seen as undesirable symptoms. The Hearing Voice Network seeks a nonmedical solution to the voices heard (and usually chemically repressed) by people who are diagnosed with psychotic diseases (Sheffield Hearing Voices Network 2010).

Splitting from Diagnosis?

Undeland and Malterud (2002) maintain that we err by seeing diagnosis as the be-all and end-all of the medical consultation. The encounter could be recast as a help-seeking interaction in which serious matters will be diagnosed and symptoms managed with reassignment, perhaps when matters brought to the doctor's attention belong in a category of care that is outside of the doctor's expertise. This is a particularly important point, if, as Stone et al. (2002)

suggest, "some diagnostic labels, particularly those that sound 'psychological,' can be perceived by patients as offensive by implying that the patients are 'putting on' or 'imagining' their symptoms or that they are 'mad.'"(p. 1449).

Stone and colleagues (2002) go further to explain that many diagnostic labels have a great ability to offend patients so labeled. They write that "although 'medically unexplained' is scientifically neutral, it had surprisingly negative connotations for patients"(p. 1449). I do not find this surprising because, as I have demonstrated above, while the label is neutral, its use is anything but. Stone calls for the restoration of the term *functional*, which, while value laden in the medical psyche, appears to be acceptable in that of the patient. The functional disorder provides "a rationale for pharmacological, behavioral, and psychological treatments aimed at restoring normal functioning . . . a useful and acceptable diagnosis for physical symptoms unexplained by disease" (Stone et al. 2002, p. 1450).

At one level, diagnosis can only be collective, because it is a classificatory tool, and classification is precisely about collecting. A diagnosis serves to label that which is the same in those that are dissimilar. This is the challenge of Ockham and the paradox of diagnosis. A disease label necessarily effaces some individual difference: a point the suffering individual will know better than anyone else.

Breaching the gap between illness and disease, and notably those symptoms that have fuzzy boundaries or multiple and inexplicable comorbidities, is often attempted through the use of technological tools. Labeling a diagnosis of exclusion requires the use of diagnostic tests to rule out all the things the diagnosis by exclusion is *not*. Demonstrating presence and absence of, or potential for, disease can also be asserted (albeit not necessarily without dispute) via diagnostic technologies. In the next chapter, I explore the role technology plays in diagnosis and how novel technologies contribute to the social framing effects on, and of, diagnosis.

CHAPTER FIVE

Driving Diagnosis

Peddlers and Pushers

> It is a most extraordinary thing, but I never read a patent medicine adver-
> tisement without being impelled to the conclusion that I am suffering
> from the particular disease therein dealt with in its most virulent form.
>
> JEROME K. JEROME (1889)

In 2005 Peter Conrad referred to new driving forces that were expanding the scope of medicine and medical authority as the "engines of medicaliza-tion." *Medicalization* is one of only a few sociological terms that have managed to integrate themselves into popular and medical parlance (Furedi 2006). The process by which medical authority or explanations infiltrate banal social ex-periences of everyday life has infused scholarly literature since the early 1970s (Zola, Conrad, and Schneider are among the seminal writers in this area). Conrad argued that while early studies of the phenomenon tended to see medical imperialism at its root, contemporary context sees a number of new players invested in promoting medical explanations for a range of conditions. Conrad's engines of medicalization emerge from the changing organization of health care, where biotechnology, consumers, and managed care organiza-tions have elbowed in on the medical profession and social movements.

Medicalization is frequently, although not invariably, enabled by diagnos-tic categories. The demand for, or proposal of, a diagnosis may be the first step in casting life's experiences as medical in nature. It is with this thought in mind that analysis of diagnosis becomes a useful activity. The fact that there is a diagnosis for this or for that condition validates the need for medical attention is warranted, justifies treatment, and consolidates an identity. It positions the condition in the medical arena and starts the ball rolling.

Disease labeling is but one of the many ways by which medicalization takes place. Further, the classification of a disease plays a substantive role outside of the identification of recognized sickness: identifying deviance, disciplining practitioners, setting research agendas, and distributing resources (Rosenberg 2002). And diagnoses hide both agendas and ideologies.

In this chapter, I review, as Conrad has done in relation to medicalization, a number of drivers of diagnosis, explicating the range of interests that can be served by the presence or awareness of particular disease entities. I then provide a case study of one particular diagnosis to demonstrate how it has become a focal point for a number of interests: namely, female hypoactive sexual desire disorder (FHSDD). Its genesis, screening, and treatment suggest the presence of powerful stakeholders and androcentric, heterosexual definitions of normal sexuality. It is not that female sexuality has not already been studied within the context of medicalization (see, for example, Tiefer 1996). This case study serves as a useful heuristic for understanding how classificatory systems describe "realities" that merit further critical scrutiny and how engines of diagnosis promote their existence.

I first explore the layers of meaning that are embodied in the diagnosis of FHSDD using some of the social framing mechanisms that Aronowitz (2008) identifies. Starting with the sociocultural framing of sexuality, and particularly female sexuality, I demonstrate how fascination with normative sexuality and the presumption of its immutable presence is unchallenged and untested in medicine. I then discuss the development of screening tools for the disease, which I present as technological mechanisms for reinforcing the presence of the diagnosis. Finally, I discuss the internal and external dynamics of consumption that constitute FHSDD as a diagnostic category. The prevalent use of the hypersexualized female in all forms of media present a fantasy of constant desire and sexual fulfillment and highlights the inadequacy of the consumer. A consumer solution is promoted by the pharmaceutical industry in the exercise of disease branding: marketing the diagnosis in order to create demand for its cure.

Engines of Diagnosis

Because, as I discuss at length in foregoing chapters, disease classification is a social activity—fluid and contingent, and reliant on knowledge, values, and social priorities—conditions become diseases at particular moments and in particular contexts. While medicine retains the ultimate authority for naming disease, there are a number of other drivers of disease labeling that we need to acknowledge.

In 1992, Payer introduced the term "disease monger" and identified a medical-industrial complex that, she argued, has a great interest in promoting the notion that the greater population is either already sick or at risk of becoming so. Her focus was on the abuse of diagnosis as a mechanism for advancing political, social, and commercial interests. She identified a range of agents that stood to benefit from the proliferation of diagnostic labels—creating a need for their products and services—including medical researchers, medical writers, health educators and promoters, the pharmaceutical and diagnostics industry, doctors, lawyers, hospitals, the courts, and insurance companies (Payer 1992).

There has since been wide-ranging critical discussion of the clinical and economic contexts of disease mongering (Payer 1992; Moynihan, Heath, and Henry 2002; Moncrieff, Hopker, and Thomas 2005; Moynihan and Cassels 2005; Wolinsky 2005; Healy 2006; Tiefer 2006; Dear and Webb 2007), with an array of definitions. Payer (1992) described mongering as "big business trying to convince essentially well people that they are sick, or slightly sick people that they are very ill." Moynihan and colleagues refer to "widening the boundaries of treatable illness in order to expand markets for those who sell and deliver treatments" (Moynihan, Heath, and Henry 2002). However, to date, sociologists have paid scant attention to the pharmaceutical industry, in great part because of the discipline's focus on the experience of illness, the secretive nature of the industry, the inadequate scientific-technical knowledge of many sociologists, and the threat of legal challenge emanating from the pharmaceutical companies (Busfield 2006; Abraham 2007).

From within a sociology of diagnosis, however, it is useful to explore and theorize about the phenomenon referred to by its critics as disease mongering, as diagnostic labels are at the fulcrum of its activities. To understand the way diagnoses are promoted by nonmedical sources requires reflection upon the pharmaceutical industry and others as well as upon the context in which diagnosis currently takes place.

The ability to promote diagnoses is facilitated by the diffusion of informational knowledge through "e-scaped" medicine as described by Nettleton and discussed in chapter 3. In this context, control over medical information shifts from doctor to a variety of other loci with manifold motivations (commercial motivation in the case of industry). The patient becomes "consumer," but not only in the commercial sense of the word. A proliferation of information and media sites are available for ingestion: direct-to-consumer advertising, online self-screening tests, patient advocacy organizations, and disease awareness campaigns. Many of these are covertly, if not overtly, propped up by the industry, which stands to gain from expanding the number of individuals under a particular diagnostic umbrella (Herxheimer 2003).

Commercial interests have an important stake in highlighting overweight as a medical diagnosis rather than a statistical deviation from normative weight. These interests go beyond the pharmaceutical industry. Fitness centers—part of a $15 billion-per-annum industry in the United States (U.S. Census Bureau 2004)—in addition to the pharmaceutical and weight-loss industries and even some practicing physicians rely heavily on promoting public belief in overweight-as-disease. Identifying obesity as a disease against which gym-goers can battle, reminding them of the ever-present "threat" of disease with body mass index charts, scales for self-monitoring, and doomsday publications about the risks of corpulence are important marketing tools both for the diagnosis of obesity and for the importance of vigilant exercise, the first justifying the second.

A large number of industries stand to benefit from the belief that overweight is a disease. This results in significant lobbying and product promotion based on the disease label (Oliver 2006). Weight reduction, muscle tone, and body shape are exceptionally strong markers of "health" to consumers (Spitzack, 1990). The gym, diet, self-help, cosmetic, pharmaceutical, fashion, publishing, and many other industries all have a financial stake in ensuring that people see their weight as problematic from a medical point of view (Jutel and Buetow, 2007).

As Campos et al. (2006) point out, even leading obesity researchers (including those who set the criteria to determine what constitutes obesity) have an economic interest in defining overweight as widely as possible, either by their partnership with the pharmaceutical industry or by their own private weight-loss clinics. Their preoccupation with overweight as disease defies evidence of lower mortality associated with overweight (BMI 25–29) than with normal weight (BMI 18.5–24.9) (Romero-Corral et al. 2006), health benefits of subcutaneous fat on hips and thighs (Nevill et al. 2006), and increase in noncancer mortality after weight loss (Nilsson et al. 2002).

Commercial influences are not the only nonmedical forces to have an interest in promoting particular diagnoses. I have used the example of "excited delirium" previously. One can well imagine what interests might be protected by the presence of this particular diagnosis. Even though the criteria for such "deliria" are far from established (Milliken 1998), attributing unexpected deaths of inmates or mental patients to disease rather than to excessive force fits comfortably with the presumed ethical behavior of the police or (in cases of restraint of the mentally ill) of care providers.

There are yet others with an incentive to promote particular diagnoses. Research teams, normally with—but sometimes without—commercial funding, are built around both legitimate and contested diseases. They attract private and public money as well as students and high-profile staff to their institutions (Burgan 2005). Similarly, politicians are often willing to engage in disease awareness campaigns to identify themselves with and exploit popular concerns. For example, the current government of New Zealand used promises about screening for prostate disease along with increased disease awareness as part of its election campaign strategy (Ryall 2007), despite recommendations from the New Zealand Guidelines Group that, even with the best possible estimates for the accuracy of the available screening tests, evidence does not support population-based screening for prostate cancer (Durham 2002).

In the remainder of this chapter, I discuss one particular diagnosis, FHSDD, whose promotion is firmly driven by a range of commercial, medical, and pharmaceutical interests. It will serve, I hope, as a poignant example of exactly what Jerome K. Jerome alludes to, perhaps in his case only humorously, in the epigraph to this chapter. The importance of diagnostic recognition is a valuable tool for those whose interests reside in public health (it *is* good to be able to recognize influenza, malaria, and chronic urinary tract infections) but also for those whose interests reside in commercial gain.

Leonore Tiefer (2006) argues that the creation and promotion of a diagnosis of "female sexual dysfunction" was influenced by three factors: a convergence of pharmaceutical companies, urologists closely associated with this industry, and media-savvy sex therapists operating within the for-profit sector. The acute interest in women's sexuality, she maintains, is linked to uncritical definitions of what constitutes normal female sexuality. It is also part of the industry's desire to expand the market for drugs like Viagra by promoting erectile dysfunction more widely than is justified (Lexchin 2006).

Female Hypoactive Sexual Desire Disorder

The matter of female libido, or at least of the association of gender with libido, is one that has preoccupied scholars for centuries. While a thorough historical survey is beyond the scope of this chapter, a bouquet of examples from various eras can still illustrate this fascination.

The often-cited myth of Tiresias, as recounted by Ovid, is a useful starting point. Tiresias was called on by the gods Jupiter and Juno to settle their argument about whether the sexual pleasure of man or woman was greatest. He was appointed to "arbitrate this jocular dispute" because he had "known both Venuses" (p. 105), having lived seven years as a woman after having been born a man. He agreed with Jupiter: women have more pleasure. Tiresias's decision was not without consequence. Juno blinded him for taking Jupiter's side. To palliate his loss of sight, Jupiter gave him the ability to know the future (Ovid 1985).

While medieval writers sought to demonstrate that organs and orgasms of men and women reflected one another, the pudenda responding like the penis during coitus, Renaissance doctors struggled to make physiological sense of female orgasm. Women were variably cast as passionless or as insatiable libidinal beasts. These polar attitudes filled medical and philosophical texts. Concern about sexual difference served as a proxy for anxiety about power and position in the public sphere (Laqueur 1990).

In Victorian times, medicine, concerned about sexual excesses, took responsibility for education about sexuality, seeking both to explain and modulate the place of desire in woman's social role and to link it with the production of healthy offspring. Some authors argued that female passion had a physiological link to conception, a position that Dr. George Napheys (1871) refuted in his late-nineteenth-century guidebook for women. He argued nonetheless that the "disposition" of the woman at the time of conception had an effect on the physical and emotional formation of the fetus and described three levels of sexuality in women: those who have generally little or no sexual feeling; a probably slightly greater group who are "more or less subject to strong passion"; and finally the "vast majority of women in whom the sexual appetite is as moderate as all other appetites" (p. 74).

Another popular medical writer, Dr. Frederick Hollick (1902), acknowledged a wide difference between the two sexes "as to the manner in which the imagination acts, owing to the difference in their characters and organization" (p. 395). He maintained that a woman, in addition to her desire to please, also has an innate sentiment of *shame* that can lead to prudery if dominant. But he also cautioned that when "the [woman's] temperament is warm, and the sexual instinct unusually strong . . . indulgence is imperatively needed, and if it cannot be had the most injurious consequences may take place, indicating the possibility of miscarriage and partial derangement" (p. 389). Dr. Mary Ries Melendy (1904), on the other hand, cautioned that in the sexual union, the wife should "not be overtaxed beyond her natural desire" should the couple be in pursuit of a high spiritual life (p. 310).

Although medical guides and handbooks addressed the matter of female sexual desire, pathologization of low libido became part of the nomenclature only in the last quarter of the twentieth century. At the beginning of that century, medicine was preoccupied with *excessive* female desire (Lunbeck 1987). It was not until 1980 that the DSM-III introduced a diagnosis of "inhibited sexual desire," a condition reported as being more common in females and described as the "persistent and pervasive inhibition of sexual desire. The judgment of inhibition is made by the clinician's taking into account factors that affect sexual desire such as age, sex, health, intensity and frequency of sexual desire, and the context of the individual's life. In actual practice this diagnosis will rarely be made unless the lack of desire is a source of distress to either the individual or his or her partner" (American Psychological Association 1980, p. 278). In 1987, the DSM-III-R recast the diagnosis as "hyposexual desire disorder," described now as "persistently or recurrently deficient or absent sexual fantasies and desire for sexual activity. The judgment of deficiency or absence is made by the clinician, taking into account factors that affect sexual functioning, such as age, sex, and the context of the person's life" (American Psychological Association 1987, p. 293). The integration of these classifications into the *International Statistical Classification of Diseases* was made somewhat later. "Inhibited sexual desire" may have figured in the 1977 ICD-9, but "hypoactive sexual desire" was not present until the ICD-10 (World Health Organization 1994).

The diagnosis of FHSDD relies on the untested assumption that all humans are endowed with demonstrable sexual urges and that their absence constitutes a pathological condition. This constitutes the fundamental structural frame to buttress the pathologization of low or nonexistent sexual desire. Masters and Johnson presented sexuality as "a drive of biologic origin deeply integrated into the condition of human existence" (qtd. in Tiefer 1996, p. 259), an important cornerstone, argues Tiefer (1996), to the development of alleged universal, biological, sexual norms.

A facile evolutionary argument supporting this assumption is that sexual urges are a biological necessity for the survival of the species. However, I use the word *facile* advisedly. That homosexuality challenges this assumption is the easiest rejoinder. While homosexuality continues to present collective challenges to a heterosexually dominant classificatory society, its nonreproductive sexual urges are no longer contained in the DSM, enunciating clearly that evolution doesn't determine what medicine chooses to classify.

As a result of this presumption, there has been little contemporary scholarly discussion of asexuality in other-than-medical terms. Being captured by medicine defuses threats to the assumptions that serve as its own foundation. Medicine is simultaneously the explanation and the discipliner. Its classificatory status announces The Way Things Are and thwarts challenges.

Kaplan (1977) is cited (in Sills et al. 2005) as one of the earliest contemporary medical researchers to discuss low sexual urge in terms of pathology, building on the interest in sexuality promoted by the work of Masters and Johnson. While she acknowledged that there is no definition of normal sexual urge, she pointed out that the sex therapy literature failed to address matters of sexual desire. She presented low urge as a problem requiring extensive therapy, and associated it with a fear of love, success, and pleasure. In the same year, Lief (1977) reported that inhibited sexual desire affected 37 percent of women in one sample and was among the most difficult sexual dysfunctions to treat. Kaplan's and Lief's interest in the issue of sexual desire as an area of therapeutic interest was enabled by the sexual liberation movement of the previous decade and its antitaboo approach to speaking of sex.

More recent medical work tends to be epidemiological in nature, confirming prevalence, incidence, and associations (always, however, emphasizing asexuality-as-pathology by confirming FHSDD as something worthy of counting). Bogaert (2004)—on the basis of preexisting data from the U.K. National Survey of Sexual Attitudes and Lifestyles—reported that one percent of the population claimed to have no sexual attraction to members of either sex.

He identified a number of associated and predictive features of asexuality, including gender (mainly women), religiosity, short stature, low education, low socioeconomic status, and poor health.

In contradistinction to this epidemiological approach to understanding asexuality, identity-based discussions take a different tack. A number of Internet groups have sprung up to offer a community for individuals who identify as asexual. Virtual communities in a general sense provide a sanctuary for alternative and stigmatized groups. Notable for their genesis in medical-lay discord about diagnosis, these groups may provide support for illnesses that medicine does not sanction (for example, see Dumit [2006] on medically unexplained symptoms, Ware [1992] on chronic fatigue, or Charland [2004] on psychiatric disorders). Or a site might reject a medically imposed diagnostic classification, seeking to redefine what medicine perceives as disease in other terms (for example, see N. Fox, Ward, and O'Rourke's work on the proanorexia movement [2005] or St-Onge, Provencher, and Ouellet on psychosis [2005]).

Scherrer (2008) studied participants in the *Asexual Visibility and Education Network* and concluded, among other things, that the language to define and the space to be asexual offered by the virtual community enabled individuals to establish an essential identity based on the absence of sexual drive. She also suggested that far less attention has been paid to asexuality than other sexual identities. Possibly as a result of its *lack* of behavior and desire, it does not draw attraction to itself and has not historically been perceived as morally or legally wrong (Bogaert 2004). Her respondents, for the most part, saw asexuality as aproblematic and naturalized it as a way of being rather than as an ontological illness.

Prause and Graham (2007) surveyed the sexuality of 1,146 students and identified 41 who identified as asexual. Of these, 63.4 percent (n = 26) were women. This subset (both men and women) attributed both benefits and drawbacks to asexuality. Benefits included avoiding intimate relationship problems, having lower health risks and social pressures, and having more free time. Drawbacks, on the other hand, were potential partner relationship problems, thinking something is wrong, negative public perception, and missing positive aspects of sex. Prause and Graham also write that asexual individuals may feel pressure to conform to the normative expectation of sexuality, a social expectation that goes beyond the control of the individual (p. 353). However, the existence of the diagnostic category, more than the lack of sexual drive itself, may provide a impetus toward identification with the illness. Because personal distress is a diagnostic criterion for FHSDD, and because distress results from worry that asexuality may be a medical problem, "the psychiatric diagnosis implying abnormality may exacerbate concerns in an asexual individual" (p. 353).

Social theory provides a perspective that challenges the pathologization of low sexual drive. In both queer and feminist theory, gender and sexuality are cast as products of social and historical context rather than of immutable biological states. Trends in social theory conceptualize these categories as plural, provisional, and situated (D. Richardson 2007), providing space for asexuality as a normal sexual preference.

The "Boston marriage," or romantic but asexual relationship between lesbians, has a long historical, albeit unacknowledged, tradition (Rothblum and Brehony 1993). Boston marriages challenge the idea that sexual activity defines relationships. Women in such relationships may or may not previously have had sexual relations between themselves or with others, but they no longer do so. In all other ways but sexual, their relationship resembles those of other lesbian couples. However, importantly, the fact of their asexuality is neither acknowledged nor broadcast. To do so would be both a political and social liability.

Naomi McCormick (in Rothblum and Brehony 1993) sees the demand for sexual pleasure as proxy for partnership as a reflection of an androcentric approach to sexuality. She writes: "It is entirely possible that many passionate female friendships enjoyed by our foremothers excluded mutual genital stimulation that people expect before categorizing a relationship as sexual or erotic. The absence of genital juxtaposition hardly drains a relationship of passion or importance" (p. 6). Jagose (2003) echoes McCormick's comments: "That such happy, well-matched couples can be so easily drawn into the jurisdiction of pathological dysfunction suggests something of the weird morphing effect of the medical/therapeutic industries on the cultural status or value of sexual desire. Not in itself necessarily desirable, desire is instead compulsory. It turns out to be banally more like the Brussels sprouts of childhood, something that is good for us and that we must have whether we like it or not."

This contextualization is muted in the assumptions underpinning the diagnosis of FHSDD. That hyposexuality is seen to be a medical problem further reinforces the taboos around discussing love without sex. Rothblum and Brehony (1993) point out that many members of the lesbian community keep their asexuality hidden because being "out" as lesbians requires them to be a model of normative lesbian relationships.

The diagnosis of FHSDD, however, disregards the historical and social context of sexuality; rather it focuses on clinical detail about attitudes toward sex. The tools of diagnosis constitute a second important framing mechanism in creating the classification itself.

Technological Change

There is a technology of FHSDD that is generative. As with the diagnosis of overweight, FHSDD cannot establish an epidemiological existence in the absence of a mechanism for assessing its presence. Powerful interests, I argue, are at play in the rush to develop the tools to establish the existence of FHSDD. Not the least of these are those that figure on the panel of the International Consensus Development Conference on Female Sexual Dysfunction, whose authoritative professional status enables its recommendations to serve as mandates. The preliminary meetings to develop the consensus conference were organized by the pharmaceutical industry and were made up of a group intentionally balanced between industry representatives and researchers either experienced or interested in working collaboratively with the industry (Moynihan 2003).

This group identified the penury of studies investigating female sexual dysfunction and the barrier presented by the absence of diagnostic frameworks (Basson et al. 2000). This call to action was supported by grants from Eli Lilly, Pentech, Pfizer, Procter and Gamble, Schering-Plough, Solvay Pharmaceuticals, TAP Pharmaceuticals, and Zonagen, just as the 19 authors of the consensus statement published from this meeting acknowledged financial or other relationships with 24 listed pharmaceutical companies. The findings of this committee were that urgent investigation was required to develop new classifications and definitions of sexual dysfunction.

The first specific instrument for assessing FHSDD or its response to various treatments was developed by Sills and colleagues and presented in 2005. Entitled the validated Sexual Interest and Desire Inventory–Female (SIDI-F), the work was both funded and copyrighted by the pharmaceutical company Boehringer Ingelheim and undertaken by its scientists (Sills et al. 2005). I detail Boehringer Ingelheim's interest in FHSDD below. Sills and his colleagues tested the 17-item rating scale on women previously diagnosed by an experienced clinician as having FHSDD. Their pilot study tested the tool on

21 participants, 9 without the disorder, and 12 with it. Sills and colleagues concluded that the scale could be used to discriminate between participants diagnosed with FHSDD and those without a clinical diagnosis, but they did not provide data from the pilot. The main study only tests women with the disorder, failing to validate sensitivity in a second independent group of patients, limiting the predictive value of the instrument.

However, a recent publication purports to supersede the SIDI-F. It is a streamlined survey tool that, its authors argue, enables nonspecialists to deal with the fraught problem of female sexual function. They describe a "growing need for simple diagnostic instruments that can be used in everyday practice by clinicians who are not specialists or experts in FSD [female sexual dysfunction]" (Clayton et al. 2009, p. 731).

The decreased sexual desire screener (DSDS) is designed to provide a simple tool that can be used by nonspecialists to diagnosis what its creators believe is a prevalent condition among women. The tool has two parts. The woman is presented with an initial set of four questions. If she answers all of these *affirmatively*, then she will answer a second set of questions. If she answers all of these *negatively* the clinician can confirm the diagnosis of FHSDD. The simplicity of the diagnostic procedure is beguiling, but both the nature of the questions and the relationship of the researchers to the commercial players in the sexual dysfunction industry give pause. The first four questions ask:

> In the past, was your level of sexual desire/interest good and satisfying to you?
> Has there been a decrease in your level of sexual desire/interest?
> Are you bothered by your decreased level of sexual desire/interest?
> Would you like your level of sexual desire/interest to increase?

A fifth question rules out other causes for the decreased sexual interest (relationship problems, systemic illness, recent obstetric or gynecological events, stress, or fatigue).

Clinicians who were not specialists or experts in the field of female sexual dysfunction then reviewed the responses and determined whether the individuals met the criteria for generalized, acquired FHSDD. Subsequently, expert clinicians conducted a standard diagnostic interview with each participant. Results of the interview and of the DSDS were then compared to validate the diagnostic ability of the tool. However, both the predictive value of this tool and the interests of the researcher who developed it must be questioned.

Predictive value reflects the probability that the tool will correctly and predictably identify the presence of the condition. This means that its use will not wrongly identify individuals without the disorder as having it. Intuitively, one senses that the first four questions of the DSDS are most likely to result in an affirmative response from many women and that the confirming set of questions will probably also result in a negative response, which would lead to a positive diagnosis. The fact that the study was validated in a population with a high prevalence of the disorder limits its ability to project across a general population.

The interests of the researcher are also worth noting. Anita Clayton is a consultant for Boehringer Ingelheim, whose relationship to FHSDD I discuss in greater depth in the next section. There I explore the dynamics of consumption, including the commodification of sexuality by pharmaceutical companies such as Boehringer Ingelheim.

Commodity Culture

When Aronowitz (2008) writes about the dynamics of consumption, he describes how the effective manipulation of consumer need has a negative effect on physical and mental health, resulting in identification of a problem as medical in nature. In the case of female sexuality, the commercial dynamic is twofold. It presents the sexual female both as commodity and as consumer. This dual burden of consumer longing and disease classification is not unprecedented. The nineteenth-century disease of kleptomania typified women as simultaneously consumers of, and consumed by, shopping (Roberts 1998).

FHSDD sustains a similar two-way street of commodity culture, in which longing for spontaneous hypersexuality is marketed and then the lack thereof is pathologized and re-presented with its concomitant cure similarly available as a consumer item. The pharmaceutical industry acts as "an engine of medicalization" (P. Conrad, 2005), transforming longing into disease. Classification (diagnosis) confirms the presumed ontological, already-always-there nature of the illness.

FHSDD's presence in commodity culture is anchored in the sale of sexuality and the public discourse that surrounds female hypersexuality in product sales. From music videos to milk advertisements, the display of the female body in sexually provocative and enticingly erotic postures is common currency (Reichert and Lambiase 2003). This positions hypersexuality as a female norm. Women are supposed to like having sex, or being sexy. Not wanting sex is not normal. So the readers of *Woman's Weekly* and *Woman's Day* follow the thousand little rules for achieving a bikini body in time for summer, simultaneously taking surveys about what turns them on, how to make *him* (not her) happy in bed, and figuring out just how often they should be having sex (if they're normal, that is) and what kind. The vexed question of "Just how often are normal people having sex?" surfaces in publications from *Glamour* to *New Scientist* and figures in self-screening tools about longevity, happiness, and relationship health.

This might be the pursuit of what Philip Cushman (1990) argues is a great consumer yearning, emerging from the transformation of the bounded, restricted Victorian self into the empty post–World War II self-contained individual. This "empty self" finds its fulfillment in consumption and acquisition, with sexuality as a prevalent theme. Glorified sexual images whose primary intent is to sell products present at the same time a mandate to be sexy, to have sex, and to desire sexual connection (Kilbourne 2003).

Sex sells magazines, clothes, cosmetics, cars, music, toothpaste, and a myriad of other items, but the reciprocal is also true: magazines, clothes, cosmetics, cars, music, and toothpaste sell sex. The fantasy of constant desire and sexual fulfillment captured in advertising serves as a perpetual reminder of the inadequacy of the consumer (Kilbourne 2003). It is a distortion of reality, presenting sexuality as it should be (at least in the eyes of able marketers), not as it is. The consumer then seeks to attain normality as it is portrayed in the imaginary. The transformation of longing into pathology is being skillfully managed by a number of players in the pharmaceutical industry, creating a second tier in the commercial dynamic that generates FHSDD as a diagnostic category (Tiefer 2006).

The story of FHSDD is infused by the efforts of the pharmaceutical industry to establish the existence of female sexual dysfunction in order to market the cure. But we'll start with the cure, to understand where the stakes are driven and how the commercial interest is promoted. It hinges on the medication Flibanserin, patented in 2006 as a treatment for FHSDD (Borsini and Evans 2006).

The primary component of Flibanserin, a compound called BIMT-17, was initially investigated as a potential antidepressant, appearing in the psychopharmacology literature for the first time in 1997 (Borsini et al. 1997), after animal studies a few years earlier (Borsini et al. 1995). The first author of these articles is a staff scientist for Boehringer Ingelheim. His work describes the substance as having a faster possible onset of therapeutic action than other established therapeutic options for depression. Later media reports about the compound reveal that during early-phase studies of its antidepressant activity, researchers monitored anticipated side effects of decreased libido and observed, rather than the expected decrease, an increase (Carey 2006). There is no published research heralding this finding. However, by December 2006, Borsini and a colleague from Canada had filed a U.S. patent application on behalf of Boehringer Ingelheim for a "method of treating female hypoactive sexual desire disorder with Flibanserin" (Borsini and Evans 2006).

Boehringer Ingelheim (BI) launched a media campaign proclaiming the importance of Flibanserin and the severity of FHSDD. On 31 October 2008, a BI press release claimed that "the largest study of its kind reveals low sexual desire is (the) most common female sexual problem" (Meyer-Kleinmann 2008a). It cites Shifren and colleagues' (2008) cross-sectional survey of 31,581 female respondents, which reported that 38.7 percent of women experienced low desire. The science behind the report seems clear. The sample size is exceptional, the p-values and confidence intervals stringent, the scale used to determine FHSDD validated.

However, closer scrutiny reveals that the study was funded by Boehringer Ingelheim, that the principle author of the paper receives consulting fees from BI, that the second and third authors were employed by BI at the time of the research, and that the remaining authors "performed work related to this article under a research contract with BI and their employer" (Shifren et al. 2008). The scale used to validate the condition was developed outside of BI, but by researchers funded by a different pharmaceutical industry player, Procter and Gamble (Derogatis et al. 2002). Procter and Gamble had a similar interest in promoting female sexual distress, given its commitment to Intrinsa, a transdermal testosterone patch for the treatment of FHSDD (Procter and Gamble Pharmaceuticals UK Ltd. 2009).

Buttressed by science generated by the pharmaceutical industry itself, Boehringer Ingelheim set forth on an awareness campaign to highlight the frequency, underdiagnosis, and consequences of FHSDD (see Meyer-Kleinmann's press release, 2008b). The company prepared an information sheet describing an unreferenced frequency of "up to one in five women" and promoting a new diagnostic tool comprising only five questions and taking less than 15 minutes to complete (Boehringer Ingelheim GmbH 2008). This is the DSDS referred to above, developed and validated by Anita Clayton and her team. As I have pointed out, Dr. Clayton is a consultant to, is funded by, and is on the advisory board of Boehringer Ingelheim. Her article reporting on the validation of the DSDS was not published until March 2009 in the *Journal of Sexual Medicine*. Boehringer Ingelheim's announcement circumvents the publication of the actual study. However, the *Journal of Sexual Medicine* is an ally of the pharmaceutical industry. It features professional endorsements on its Web site from Pfizer and Bayer (www.wiley.com/bw/journal .asp?ref=1743-6095) and no others.

Of course, Clayton is not the only researcher in this area with strong ties to industry. The medical opinion leaders in the discussion of FHSDD are, for the most part, affiliated with Boehringer Ingelheim or with related industrial players. Most of the consensus writers in 1999, who originally set the scene, and the authors of recent reviews of the condition and the expert clinicians developing tools have an affiliation with Boehringer Ingelheim either through funding of the studies being reported or in a consultant role (Shifren;[1] Clayton;[2] Sills, Wunderlich, Pyke, and Segraves;[3] and so on). Boehringer Ingelheim is not alone in funding the tools and providing cures for female sexual dysfunction. I have mentioned Procter and Gamble but Pfizer (and perhaps others) also have a vested interest in the development of other treatments for female sexual dysfunction.

The consumer dynamic is clearly complex. It involves an initial and pervasive representation to the consumer of sexuality as a means of escape from the real conditions of existence. Sexuality circulates as an attainable promise that must be eternally deferred for the promise to be unendingly remade (Brady 2007). On one hand, consumer culture is based on perpetuating feelings of sexual inadequacy; on the other, the industry has recognized an opportunity for exploitation and has designed and presented a panacea, also for sale.

Discussion

Moving away, for a moment, from FHSDD, we should consider that this is neither the first nor the only way in which women's putative diseases have reflected social understandings about the way women should be. Tacit cultural knowledge about the nature of women and of femininity figures is widely captured in the guise of objective, scientific fact. From the ancient Greeks, who claimed that hysteria was caused by a lack of sexual intercourse (Rodin 1992), to Victorian doctors, who maintained that a woman's menses prevented her from engaging in physical or intellectual activity (Vertinsky 1994), it has been common practice throughout the history of women's diseases to assert that symptoms are related to women's sexuality and conformity (or lack thereof) to prescribed social roles.

Premenstrual syndrome emerges from Hippocrates's hysteria, transformed along the way by the logic of the *Malleus Maleficarum* (which held that women were prone to alliances with the Devil) and by Renaissance thinkers who envisioned hysteria as a neurological disease (Rodin 1992). In 1931, the condition was first delineated in a formal, clinical context as "premenstrual tension" (Rodin 1992, p. 49). Emotional symptoms of premenstrual tension included nervousness, irritability, depression, and generalized emotional tension. "Premenstrual syndrome" was coined in 1953. Despite the inability of researchers to provide adequate scientific proof linking the stated emotional qualities to PMS, the link has remained in medical discourse (Rodin 1992).

Diseases linked to the female menstrual cycle have a controversial recent history. The DSM-III-R included "Late luteal phase dysphoric disorder," or LLPDD, defined as a psychiatric disorder characterized by recurrent, cyclic periods of dysphoria corresponding with the menstrual cycle. Other physical and emotional symptoms associated with PMS were not included, and according to the DSM-III-R, only 5 percent of those with PMS would qualify as having LLPDD.

Those in support of including LLPDD in the DSM argued that it would stimulate research and would encourage doctors to treat women's complaints more seriously. Opponents countered that women would be inappropriately diagnosed as mentally ill, or alternatively, women could use the diagnosis to justify criminal behavior (Rodin 1992). The Committee on Women of the American Psychiatric Association argued that even a carefully worded definition of the disease could be misconstrued so that all menstruating women could be dismissed as "crazy " (Lorber and Moore 2002). How the condition could be defined in classification documents hinged upon how it was understood both by those attempting to classify it and those protesting its classification as disease. Were these variations in women's mood presumed to be linked to the menstrual cycle the result of hormonal, social, or gynecological factors? Or were they, as opponents argued, simply evidence of normal physiology? The failure to agree upon how PMS could be typified as a disease resulted in a call for more research, a compromise outcome that frustrated those who had hoped to exclude PMS from the DSM altogether (Lorber and Moore 2002).[4]

Perhaps an even more controversial women's diagnosis is the gendered "self-depreciating personality disorder," originally to be called "masochist personality disorder" (MPD). According to the draft for the DSM-III-R, women who have MPD make no demands on others, are self-sacrificing, are uncomfortable with success and recognition, feel unworthy, and neglect their own pleasure for that of others (Kutchins and Kirk 1997). Feminist groups argued that MPD would be used to describe women who were in abusive relationships. The features of this proposed diagnosis have been lauded social characteristics of the ideal woman, creating, paradoxically, a disease out of heroic femininity. Literary examples of people with MPD would astound readers of women's fiction: Beth in *Little Women*, Melanie in *Gone with the Wind*, Sara in *The Little Princess*, and Mary in the *Little House* series were held as sainted examples of proper womanhood, as they self-effaced before all, generous, unflinching, and probably—according to these diagnostic criteria—ill. The neoliberal context of self-interest, self-promotion, and individual self-realization does not celebrate these visions of femininity but promotes a discourse of freedom and flexibility.

This would be a case of what Gaines (1992) describes as the "voice of classification": valuing self-control and self-mastery, privileging an ideal gender (male), ethnicity (German Protestant), and age (adult) over others. Because women do not fit into the idealized self, they are the focus of considerable attention in the DSM.

FHSDD is a vivid example of how the convergence of social circumstances leads first to the identification of a particular condition as problematic and second to its embodiment in a diagnostic framework. In this case, the disease category is relatively transparent but no less controlling. It would be simplistic to argue that FHSDD is simply the creation of the pharmaceutical industry, a perfect example of disease mongering. Without minimizing the role of the industry in the promotion and expansion of this diagnosis, I maintain that the industry cannot conjure a classification out of thin air.

A particular social context must provide the backdrop for the disease branding that Boehringer Ingelheim is undertaking with FHSDD. In this case, an age-old angst over women's sexuality, overlaid by the commodification of sexuality, provides a context within which the industry can drive for public and professional recognition of the disorder rather than leaving it hidden in the pages of the DSM or the ICD, pulled out and dusted off for only the odd idiosyncratic case. In the case of FHSDD, the pharmaceutical industry alone could not make the diagnosis a wider concern if, for example, female sexuality were still generally taken as woman's duty to her spouse and nation. Imagine for a moment if those who provided advice to young married women still believed today, as J. A. Stewart did in 1814 when providing "advice previous to matrimony," that "the tumult of passion will necessarily subside" (J. Stewart 1814, p. 540). The first questions of Clayton's DSDS screening tool would, in that context, make no sense. Rather than capturing a picture of pathology, they would be describing the normal state of affairs: yes, my level of desire used to be good; yes, my level desire is lower than it was; yes, my passion has subsided.

While Stewart did not incriminate passion as deviant, by the turn of the next century, female hypersexuality figured large in psychiatric medicine as an ailment. Psychiatrists used the term "psychopathic" to describe women who engaged in sexual activity beyond the bounds of what genteel society felt was moral (Lunbeck 1987). Such women were cast as sexual predators who sought to entrap young men through their "uncontrolled sex impulses," in stark contrast with the medical concern over female sexuality today.

For FHSDD to exist, sexuality must be a desired female attribute, and women must be capable of indulging their impulses without recrimination. Perpetual reminders of both of these factors serve to reposition the self as one who can have FHSDD. The transformation from the dangerous Victorian self, whose sexual and aggressive impulses had to be controlled by state and church, to the self-expressive, consuming, and indulgent self is an important prerequisite to any commercial strategy using inadequate sexuality as foundation (Cushman 1990). Cushman rightly maintains that understanding the configuration of the self and its temporal context provides insights on "the illnesses that plague it, and the activities responsible for healing it"(p. 600).

Knowing what consumers feel and believe is an important foundation to any branding campaign, and Boehringer Ingelheim's intimate involvement in the promotion, identification, and cure of FHSDD is an exercise in disease branding.[5] This approach doesn't market the therapy but rather the awareness of the condition that the therapy is supposed to cure. An effective disease-branding strategy results in sufficient public awareness for intervention no longer to be required: the patient and doctor are vigilant monitors of the potential for diagnosis (Parry 2007).

Understanding the diagnosis and its genesis provides another angle for understanding the medicalization of women's sexuality. First, the mechanisms that frame this diagnostic label, as described above, are firmly grounded in a social context that must be acknowledged. The diagnosis enables the expansion of medical authority and its agents (or "engines"). Second, the FHSDD label fulfils the potent social roles one expects of a diagnosis. It legitimizes deviance, defines normality, creates identity, and enables access to treatment (Jutel 2010a). Finally, however, it reinforces an inadequately challenged combination of assumptions and observations about sexual function that consequently serve as a basis for commercial exploitation and disease promotion.

CHAPTER SIX

"There Is Nothing So Small as to Escape Our Inquiry"

Technologies of Diagnosis

> Who is able by seeing the blood to divine whether it be an intermittent or a continuall feavor, whether a dysentery or haemoptoe the patient is sick of, and what sensible fault does often appear in that bloud in which nature does sometimes expel the cause of a disease, and give present ease by a critical haemorrhagia wherein the bloud very often looks as florid and as well conditioned as any that flows in the veins of the most healthy man living?   JOHN LOCKE (IN DEWHURST 1966)

John Locke was an empiricist and a skeptic. He firmly believed that medicine could advance only through experience and observation (Wolfe 1961). His medicine was typified by observed phenomena, external resemblances, and practical classification of diseases and their treatments. He maintained that the warrant of medicine was to save men from death, not to engage in the discovery of causes. In his view, looking for causes was a luxurious intellectual pursuit that did little to serve mankind. Locke considered this a form of speculation that did not aid practice. His objections to the study of the cause of disease may be grounded in the technological limitations of his era. He wrote, "Nature performs all her operations on the body by parts so minute and insensible that I thinke noe body will ever hope or pretend, even by the assistance of glasses . . . , to come to a sight of them" (qtd. in Wolfe 1961, p. 213).

Locke's reluctance to use technology in medical research bears little resemblance to contemporary approaches to health and illness. Modern approaches highlight the powerful capacity of technology to contribute to the empirical: to perceive that which the naked eye—or the phenomenon-experiencing subject—cannot. We are accustomed to the blood test, the urine culture, or the x-ray as a means of confirming "what we've got." We might even be suspicious of the clinician who delivers a diagnosis with minimal technological support, who draws on palpation, auscultation, patient account, or other clinical observations to arrive at a conclusion. "How does he know it's not something else?"

This is not the first time in the pages of this book that technology has surfaced as an actor in diagnosis. I have touched on the diagnostic role of technology in previous chapters and have noted that the introduction of classificatory categories (new diagnoses) is contingent on technological advancement, just as the act of diagnosis may rely on and promote technology in preference to clinical observation and the patient's own report.

Technology plays an increasingly important role in Western medicine. Since the mid-1980s, medicine has changed and extended its authority through an increasingly technoscientific formulation (Clarke et al. 2003). Risk is monitored; medical knowledges are produced and consumed differently; information is standardized, quantified, scrutinized, and analyzed; identities are re-created along molecular and genetic lines (Clarke et al. 2003). Technology establishes, monitors, recognizes, and treats diseases. In the following pages, I examine some of the ways in which technology fulfils these tasks.

Technology and Diagnostic Categories

As in the case of Alzheimer disease and the discovery of neurofibrillary tangles discussed in chapter 4, technology is often at the base of what medicine is capable of defining as illness. Recall that it was advanced staining techniques that enabled Alzheimer to distinguish this particular form of cognitive decline from the more mundane senility of old age. Technological advances enable the recognition of many other diagnostic categories. In sickle-cell anemia, for example, diagnostic labeling could never have taken place without the ability to create a laboratory profile of human blood, viewing sickle-shaped red blood cells on glass slides. The disease itself presented with varying clinical pictures but was not clearly distinguishable from other anemias, parasitic ailments, and syphilis. It was the microscopic profile of the "sickling" cell that enabled the creation of a new diagnosis. The blood smear, more than the clinical presentation, was at the heart of this diagnosis, coined in 1922 by Verne Mason (Feldman and Tauber 1997). Of course, in the absence of microscopy, the distinction between the sickle-shaped cell and other anemias was not conceivable.[1]

Examples such as this abound. What science and technology are able to capture influences what medicine is able to describe. Microbiology, virology, and genetics have all contributed to framing new diagnoses and effacing others. Consumption's transformation to tuberculosis was grounded in microscopy, anchored by the 1882 isolation of the tubercle bacillus by Robert Koch (Daniel 2006),[2] while multiple sclerosis was slowly extirpated from rheumatic disease, constitutional weakness, and paralysis agitans by manual examination of the brain and spinal cord in postmortem examination (Murray 2005).

We don't know what diseases lurk around the corner, what microbe or genetic modification concealed to our eye today will be revealed by technology tomorrow, or similarly, which of the diseases we firmly believe in today will have a completely different form and defining characteristics in a decade or two. The advancement of genetics, proteomics, and molecular profiling progressively exposes new and unexpected diagnoses. What was once simply breast cancer is now differentiated, not just on size and grade of the tumor, menopausal status of the patient, nodal involvement, or cell type, but also on estrogen or progesterone receptivity and differential gene expression.

Technology has changed our thinking about cancer diagnoses and treatment, with particular gene profiles relating to better or worse prognoses (Sotiriou et al. 2003). Here, Ockham's razor is finely honed, as genomics and proteomics seek to identify the multiplicity of variations present in individual patients and then to tailor treatment at the molecular level. Ockham's principle was that groups of things should not be split any more than necessary. However, therapeutic necessity seeks narrow classifications: the greater the specificity of the diagnosis, the more tailored the treatment and the more effective the outcome. Such specificity is clearly enabled by technologically.

Yet technology is not independent in identifying what counts as disease. Technologies are themselves products of their own cultural moment (Wailoo 1997). As Wailoo documents, notably in reference to hematology, disease construction owes much to the technologies of medicine but not in isolation from medical and cultural context.

The example of chlorosis, a disease that slowly faded from both medical and public repertories at the turn of the twentieth century, provides a useful case in point. Initially presented in social terms, chlorosis was the disease of the delicate woman. It occurred in the overtaxed and the understimulated, the malnourished and the overnourished, the working and leisure classes. This disease presented in young women as a pallor that was so extreme as to lend a greenish tinge to the complexion. It was accompanied by tachycardia, shortness of breath, amenorrhea, and gastric difficulties. Wailoo describes three narratives that framed chlorosis and ultimately brought about its demise. The first saw the genesis of the disease in the biological failure of the young woman to adjust to modern society and in society's failure to recognize feminine frailty. The concordant treatment involved careful improvements in physical activity, reduction of external stresses, nourishing food, frequent bowel movements, and ample rest. The second narrative departed from the gender-centered conception to recast chlorosis technologically, according to hematological profile. The appearance of the chlorotic hemocyte anchored new explanations for the illness. A pale red blood cell visible in the chlorotic patient provided a technological transformation from social to hematological, with "hypochromic anemia" taking the place of chlorosis. Finally, a pharmaceutical approach, born of therapeutic reductionism, anchored chlorosis in the technology of iron metabolism, seeing the green sickness in terms of iron-deficiency anemia, and casting a new identity for the nineteenth-century disease. For Wailoo, it is the interaction of technologies with medicine and cultural values that shaped chlorosis's many identities as well as their demise.

Technology is thus not only contained in instrumentation and new forms of imaging or immune assaying but is also embedded in approaches to knowledge. The science of an era enables some diagnoses and eliminates others. Humoral theory explained disease by the influence of heat, cold, dryness, and moisture on the body. Heat induced relaxation, and cold induced restriction of minute fibers of which the body was believed to be constituted (G. Miller 1962). This could result in diseases such as melancholia. This incapacitating state of sadness, fearfulness, and fatigue was attributed to (and etymologically means) "black bile." It was associated with an excess of coldness and dryness (S. Jackson 1978).

Contemporary diagnostic conceptualization has a similar impact on what can be seen as disease. This "technoscientization," as Clarke and her colleagues have called it, includes the domination of evidence-based medicine in conceptualizing disease. The evidence-based medicine "paradigm" (often now referred to as a "cause" or a "movement") is recent, launched in 1992 by a seminal article published in the *Journal of the American Medical Association* and written by the Evidence-Based Medicine Working Group, under the chair of Gordon Guyatt. Its recent origins could be traced to Archie Cochrane's 1972 diatribe on effectiveness and efficiency. There, he lamented the absence of measurement of effectiveness of medical interventions and described the randomized controlled trial as a tool for "open[ing] up the new world of evaluation and control" (p. 433) and perhaps saving the national health service (Cochrane 1989).

Evidence-based medicine is grounded in a statistical model of medicine, which applies formal rules of evidence for evaluating research literature, and in principles of epidemiology guiding day-to-day clinical practice (Evidence-Based Medicine Working Group 1992). The central tenet of evidence-based medicine is the hierarchy of evidence, which privileges certain kinds of information over others. As postulated by the Evidence-Based Medicine Working Group, "systematic attempts to record observations in a reproducible and unbiased fashion markedly increase the confidence one can have in knowledge about patient prognosis, the value of diagnostic tests, and the efficacy of treatment. In the absence of systematic observation one must be cautious in the interpretation of information derived from clinical experience and intuition, for it may at times be misleading" (p. 2421).

One important result of the hierarchy of evidence that accompanies evidence-based medicine (EBM) is the way in which it transforms what *counts* as disease. Meta-analysis and randomized controlled trials are the highest levels of evidence on the hierarchy and elbow other forms of knowledge out of the way. Things that can be counted and standardized (and therefore evaluated as variables, tested against controls, and statistically synthesized) gain supremacy. Morse has argued that EBM is a politics of ignorance—myopic and exclusionary—that uses Cochrane's standards for evaluating funding for all forms of research. He claims it's a fine sieve that ends up funding drug trials by the powerful and relegating qualitative researchers who are unable to access funds, credibility, and, importantly, power (Morse 2006). As Clarke and colleagues (2003) point out, the information required by EBM (objectified, sanitized, computerized and statistically analyzed) prevents the clinician from taking the individual body into account. In my often-cited example of overweight, EBM plays an important role in its transformation from simple descriptive adjective to disease. Weight is quantitative and imparts implied neutrality (in contrast to the presumed biased subjectivity of self-reported activity or diet), which allows the scales to serve as a proxy measure of wellness, creating a convenient mechanism for understanding corpulence.

Therapeutic technology also frames diagnostic categories. Blaxter (1978) noted that the existence of effective treatment refines the understanding of the conditions for which treatment is intended. Wailoo's (1997) discussion of hematological disorders demonstrates the degree to which response to treatment framed diagnostic groups. The administration of liver extracts for pernicious anemia resulted in such dramatic response that treatment effect determined how patients would be classified. Wailoo calls the treatment a diagnostic tool, "structuring not only medical practice and research, but medical thinking about the identity of the disease" (p. 124). Those cases that did not respond to liver extract were reclassified as "atypical" or "anomalous."

As an extension of this consideration of therapy-as-diagnosis, I reflect back to the discussion of the engines of diagnosis and consider the technological role of pharmaceutical industry interests in the identification of diseases. Returning to female hypoactive sexual desire disorder, we can see how clinical trials of BIMT-17 as an antidepressant resulted in improved libido in the female participants. This accidental finding is similar to what researchers found when they initially trialed what was to become Viagra. The substance was being tested to determine its efficacy in the reduction of angina and was found to lead to a side effect of penile erection in some subjects (Ban 2006). That this discovery coincided with the "discovery" of erectile dysfunction as a debilitating condition affecting more than 40 percent of U.S. men is linked closely to the potential market this putative therapeutic agent can satisfy (Lexchin 2006). The success of the trials of Flibanserin (BIMT-17) provides a similar technological frame for confirming the presence of FHSDD.

Technology and the Diagnostic Process

Technology tells us things about illness and disease that count for more than what we can say ourselves. In the diagnostic process, technological perspectives are often privileged over the subjective lived experience of the lay person. In the next few paragraphs I take you on a personal journey to illustrate this point.

On a Thursday, one week in May, I made an appointment to see my GP, Dr. C. When he came to the waiting room to bring me back to his office, we exchanged the regular preexamination banter. "So, how are you doing?" he asked with an appropriate amount of concern in his voice. "Absolutely fantastic! Cured!" I chirruped as we walked into his rooms. He looked at me, mildly confused at this positive response. I had been a regular visitor to his office since late January, and the previous week I had been one of his daily call-back patients. I had initially presented with an enigmatic and progressively incapacitating cough. Although I was basically well, the cough was so debilitating that I had been unable to lecture, run, sleep—all those things that are part of my daily life. I had almost canceled the overseas trip I had planned for later that month. In the doctor's office, other patients would move to the other side of the waiting room when they heard me hack; I certainly couldn't inflict myself on airline passengers. I probably would have been too uncomfortable to make the long trip anyway.

My x-ray and blood tests had been normal. However, a banal *haemophilus* (which may occur as normal flora of the nose and pharynx, but which may also cause illness in the presence of immunosuppression) was initially present in my sputum. I was prescribed antibiotics, with no relenting of the symptoms. A more refined serology test showed exposure (not infection), possibly historical, to pertussis (whooping cough), and a further course of antibiotics was undertaken, with similarly disappointing results. I continued to hack away. Sputum cultures and blood tests were all normal, but I remained ill. Finally, a locum who didn't know me from Adam and probably just wanted me out of his hair threw diagnostic concern out the window. He prescribed a simple symptomatic treatment of inhaled and oral anti-inflammatory medication, and my cough resolved in a matter of few short hours. There was no diagnosis to label my affliction, but I was better.

Dr. C put his head in his hands as he thought about the trajectory. "I can't believe I didn't try that sooner," he said, embarrassed that I could be "fixed" so easily, and yet it had taken almost five months to figure it out. But it was clear to me, as I said to him, that this specific diagnostic journey was a poignant example of a general trend in medicine, where we subordinate the symptom to the disease and promote the objectivity of science and its associated technological tools to interpret illness.

Leder (1990) laments medicine's current "flight from interpretation" in favor of a form of "immediate apprehension from which hermeneutical subjectivity has been expunged" (p. 20)—in other words, contemporary medicine's reliance on "objective" tests and images such as laboratory values, radiological images, and the like. He underlines the rise of technology in the diagnostic process. The appeal of transparent, objective, and irrefutable information about the body—detached from both patient and doctor—intervenes to a fault in the diagnostic process.

In addition to overreliance on what Leder terms the "instrumental," or the purified objectivity of the laboratory finding, a semiotic approach to symptoms further explains the clinical inefficacy of this case. Semiotics is the linguistic study of signs. Simplistically, words (signifiers) represent mental concepts and objects (signifieds). According to Foucault (1963), this semiotic transformation took place in the early nineteenth century with the birth of clinical medicine. Where previously the symptom was the focus of medical practice, now it became a signifier of pathology, the first sign of disease. He wrote, "Cough, fever, stitch and respiratory difficulties are not pleurisy, which is itself never revealed to the senses . . . but they constitute its essential symptoms" (p. 89). Foucault argued that semiotic theory provides an understanding of clinical observation. The constellation of symptoms point invariably to an underlying disease process. As he explained, "the very heart of illness will give itself up completely in the intelligible syntax of the signifier" (p. 91).

In this context, the symptom is assumed to contain clarity and logic with respect to the disease that necessarily creates it. No longer does the symptom function as an individual phenomenon. Rather, it provides an important link to interiority and to the disease that is otherwise unseen. The clinician is a detective working to uncover the link between signifier and disease. In my own case described above, the pursuit of the hidden condition—autoimmune lung disease or infectious process—was the focus of the interpretive analysis of the abnormal cough. As the doctors delved, they uncovered possible causal agents, but the appropriate treatment resulted in no change in symptoms, belying the relationship between the presumed cause and the clinical complaint. The therapeutic intensity waned with the lack of evidence of disease, even as the cough worsened. The doctors advised me to "wait" or "see how things go," with a reduced sense of immediacy over treatment despite the deterioration in my sense of wellness. I was incapacitated, unable to engage in my normal activities of daily living, and exhausted from unremitting bouts of coughing consuming me by day and waking me and my husband by night.

The fact that my affliction was not a disease was simultaneously a relief and a frustration. On one hand, it was reassuring that there was no evidence of sarcoidosis, tuberculosis, infection, or malignancy. On the other, because the explanation for my discomfort could not be shown by an objectively visible test result confirming a known disease, my doctors overlooked symptomatic management. One might argue that these doctors failed in their task, not thinking to provide somatic relief, but I believe they acted coherently within a semiotic disease model, in which the symptom is the projection of disease. If the symptom is principally a sign or predictor of an underlying process, it is subordinated to the presumed cause and cannot feature as a clinical entity of its own. Treatment then targets the cause as opposed to the complaint, making the notion of symptomatic treatment incoherent and pushing the doctor toward the irrefutable instrumental (technological) evidence of the disease.

Diagnostic coherence guides clinical interpretation, writes Leder. It is the way in which the doctor generates provisional diagnoses, tests possible explanations, asks pertinent questions, and prevents each patient encounter from being a start-from-the-beginning random treasure hunt. The more familiar the doctor is with the values and understandings contained in this paradigm, the better will be the potential for effective care. Recognizing the semiotic importance accorded the symptom allows the doctor to diagnose soundly, as well as to determine what to do in the absence of identifiable illness.

Complaints without apparent cause are troublesome. They not only fail to signify disease but frustrate patient and doctor alike. A skeptical clinician may doubt the experiential account of the patient, while a compassionate one may feel impotent and inadequate. The lack of explanation is a threat to medical competence, and suffering can be augmented by anxiety of uncertainty. The physical nature of the complaint may be doubted and, in the absence of diagnosis, may be relegated to the realm of the psychiatric. Indeed, recommendations around medically unexplained symptoms focus on patient emotional management: demonstrating belief in the patient's complaint; giving a positive explanation, including psychological factors; and recommending a return to normal life, as well as cognitive behavioral therapy or antidepressants (Sharpe 2002).

My cough provides an effective illustration of the limitation of this approach. One might argue that this case has a different status than many cases of non-disease-related symptoms, because the clinical complaint is verifiable by the doctor, can be observed and assessed, and could only be feigned with difficulty (unlike complaints of "dizziness," "fatigue," or "pain," whose physical presence cannot be witnessed as easily by the clinician). Here the interpretive challenge was not hindered by any disagreement over what had pushed me to see the doctor. What I felt and reported was never denied by the GP or by the specialist, nor did they redefine the narrative as being either nonmedical or nonphysical.

Leder (1990) refers to the "sovereignty of the machine" and the "purified objectivity" conveyed by what he calls "instrumental texts," which we could perhaps call in the context of this chapter "technological texts." In this case, the sputum and serology reports misled, and the duration of patient suffering was consequently unreasonably prolonged. The doctors sought to treat the disease rather than the patient. The cough was simply a cough. Anti-inflammatory treatment made it go away.

This is what Leder describes as a pursuit of objective reality and unambiguous results, leading the clinician away from the patient. "The person-as-ill tends to disappear from view when the focus is placed exclusively on certain secondary and tertiary texts. . . . In its attempt to expunge interpretive subjectivity, modern medicine thus threatens to expunge the subject" (pp. 20–21).

The reliance on diagnostic imaging, in the United States at least, is fueled by financial imperative. Profit is embedded in procedures rather than in clinical assessment. A steady increase in the prescription of, and reimbursement for, diagnostic imaging emerges from this principle. With traditional sources of income for doctors being "squeezed," American doctors have been led to seek other revenue streams, among which diagnostic testing features prominently. The cost of radiological imaging is covered by Medicare and therefore renders the use of x-ray, CT, and MRI attractive to the primary-care physician. A kind of medical entrepreneurship has resulted in almost a quarter of MRI machines being owned by nonradiologist physicians, who gain a return on investment by the high volume of images they generate (Berlin and Berlin 2005).

Screening

There is another side to this story. Up to this point I have considered only the person-as-ill whose illness doesn't find expression in the objective technology of science. But just as salient is the person-as-well whose wellness is refuted by objective findings. David Armstrong's powerful article "The Rise of Surveillance Medicine" (1995) depicts a medicine concerned with detecting illness before the individual's health is even affected. It is a medicine in which symptoms are not coterminous with disease. Rather, disease is seen as a silent, unobtrusive potentiality, ready to rear its ugly head in the seemingly healthy when least expected. In surveillance medicine, illness is a complicated set of interrelated states, from apparent healthiness to precursor signs and finally to overt symptoms of recognized disease.

The idea that ostensibly healthy individuals should subject themselves to medical scrutiny, even in the absence of disease symptoms, dates well back, to at least the mid-nineteenth century. Horace Dobell, in 1861, posited that even well people should have periodic health examinations, because diseases, he believed, were preceded by a state of low health that could provide an opportune window for early treatment (Han 1997). Similarly, George Gould, some years later, suggested that "personal biological examinations" would help doctors both prevent and treat disease before it occurred (Han 1997).

The screening of surveillance medicine extends the diagnostic power to a space *before* disease. The risk factors "are pointers to a potential, yet unformed, eventuality" (Armstrong 1995, p. 402). As such, both screening and diagnostic events contain a similar transformative power. The abnormal cells, the elevated laboratory values, the unexpected blip on the electrocardiogram—all provide the rationale for treatment or lifestyle modification in one who feels him- or herself to be well.

Surrogate Markers

Prominent in screening tests are surrogate markers and endpoints. A surrogate marker is a laboratory test results that has a theoretical link with the disease one is trying to detect and prevent. For example, cholesterol, blood pressure, coronary vessel diameter, and left ventricular hypertrophy are among the surrogate markers for heart attacks and heart failure, but none of these is a true clinical endpoint or evidence of the disease. Each (the last two on the list, far more markedly than the preceding examples) is linked to diagnosis of the clinical event (heart disease) and points toward that event, but in different degrees. The marker captures evidence of the process that is thought to underlie the disease (Temple 1999). High levels of cholesterol can lead to atherosclerosis, which in turn can lead to reduced coronary vessel diameter, and ultimately to myocardial infarction. In principle, then, each of these markers might be a predictor or indicator of the potential for the clinical outcome one is attempting to prevent. The principle is clear, and the FDA requires that surrogate markers be "reasonably likely" to predict clinical benefit when they are used as evidence of clinical utility. However, in practice, surrogate markers are problematic.

The use of surrogate markers in health screening is a clear nod to the never-truly-healthy nature of human subjects. Further, their use in clinical research is often more useful for marketing than it is valid for patient outcomes (Grimes and Schulz 2005; Freemantle and Calvert 2007). Using surrogate as opposed to clinical endpoints is fraught: medications that are designed to reduce cholesterol levels in order to decrease the potential for cardiovascular disease do not necessarily achieve their goal. As one example, in clinical trials, statin drugs (ezetimibe and simvastatin) lowered serum cholesterol but did not slow the development of heart disease (atherosclerosis) in patients (Kastelein et al. 2008), their putative role.

At a population level, it's easy to see that the risk approach embedded in surrogate markers has limitations. For example, European cardiovascular guidelines use markers that would classify most adult Norwegians at high risk, despite Norway's having one of the world's longest-living and healthiest populations (Getz et al. 2005).

Routine screening seeks to find evidence of disease in a patient who is presenting for what may be unrelated, and possibly not even clinical, reasons. While there has been a rise in screening as part of health assessment, there is significant debate about its claimed benefits. Black (2000) argues that detecting subclinical conditions (pseudodiseases), which would otherwise have gone to the grave with the patient (while not being the cause of death), can result in anxiety, unnecessary treatment, complications, and even actual death. Overdiagnosis, he asserts, is a direct result of unnecessary screening, which does not in fact reduce disease-specific mortality. Treating pseudodisease does not improve the odds of those who have real disease. In the case of the Mayo Lung Project, which tested the effectiveness of intensive screening for lung cancer against the standard nonscreening approach, mortality from lung cancer was actually *higher* in the screened group than in the control. This is probably due to the fact that imaging techniques can identify a range of abnormal nodules of unknown clinical significance (Marcus et al. 2006).

Screening for disease is practiced with religious fervor, according to Howard Brody (2006), but not always with the acquiescence of the patient. On the surface, it would hardly seem problematic to detect what might be silent for now but disease later. Yet there are many unintended consequences of screening that we should consider, including overtreatment, longer morbidity for cases where the prognosis is unaltered by the early diagnosis, false negative results, and of course, morbidity from diagnostic testing and overzealous treatment, particularly in those with false positive results (Jepson 2006).

Political uses of screening are worth noting. In a recent New Zealand election, an important plank of the incoming government's platform was based on the commonsense notion that because breast cancer screening was an established public health initiative, prostate cancer screening should be similarly promoted for all men. The vote-generating discourse around this initiative was that men were a neglected underclass who *deserved* screening, despite medical evidence pointing to the important morbidities of prostate cancer screening (Black 2000).

Confirming the value of such approaches is possibly the fact that popular belief, in the United States at least, and as confirmed by Schwartz and colleagues' 2004 study, is that screening is "almost always a good idea," even if it does not lead to effective treatment or the screening reveals pseudodisease (L. Schwartz et al. 2004). An exaggerated sense of disease risk, the commercial marketing of screening devices and approaches, and inadequate public exploration of how and when screening contributes to well-being are probably at the root of these beliefs (L. Schwartz et al. 2004).

Other markers serve a quite different purpose and, instead of stigmatizing, legitimize illness experiences. A case in point is the genetic markers observed in veterans of nuclear testing. One cohort of nuclear test veterans in 1957 observed as many as nine nuclear detonations in the mid-Pacific Ocean (at Kiribati, Malden Island, and Christmas Island). A number of the veterans who witnessed these detonations have reported a range of medically unexplained symptoms: genetic disorders among their offspring and increased incidence of multiple myeloma, gastric and respiratory disorders, and arthritis. The claims made by these veterans have been difficult to prove, as much of the documentary evidence of their exposure is controlled by the parties the veterans claim are culpable: the British and New Zealand navies (Trundle 2010).

Genetic testing of 50 individuals from within this group compared with results for 50 matched controls has demonstrated chromosomal damage (Wahab et al. 2008). Translocation and extraordinarily complex chromosomal rearrangements such as those viewed in these tests are generally suggestive of radiation exposure. These biological markers (chromosome translocation frequency) became an important evidentiary tool for those servicemen seeking compensation for themselves and their families on the basis of radiation to which they were exposed during the tests. Here, the genetic marker is not a stigmata, as in the preceding examples, but a tangible indication of liability, according to these veterans. It legitimizes their suffering and their anxieties and opens the way for compensation.

Other markers may be used in occupational health to identify early effects of toxic agents in the body (exposure) or individual predispositions to be more or less favorably affected by chemical exposure (susceptibility). Although such monitoring is part of many occupational health and safety strategies, it raises ethical concerns about workers' well-being, including job loss, stigmatization, reassignment, and insurance or mortgage ineligibility (Caux et al. 2007).

Genetic Discrimination

Disease potential is a salient means of social control and is amplified by the ever-expanding technical access to new screening tools. Lippman (1991) describes how genetic risk in particular captures an increasingly wider array of social concerns: "Using the metaphor of blueprints, with genes and DNA fragments presented as a set of instructions, the dominant discourse describing the human condition is reductionist, emphasizing genetic determination. It promotes scientific control of the body, individualizes health problems and situates individuals increasingly according to their genes. Through this discourse, which is beginning seriously to threaten other narratives, clinical and research geneticists and their colleagues are conditioning how we view, name and propose to manage a whole host of disorders and disabilities. Though it is only one conceptual model, 'genetics' is increasingly identified as *the* way to reveal and explain health and disease, normality and abnormality" (p. 18).

Genetic screening becomes a modern/countermodern form of biological determinism, which describes the supposed social risk presented by this or that particular profile, giving individuals the potential to respond to their future and plan healthy offspring. However, the genetic movement has difficulty shifting its eugenic roots (Kerr and Cunningham-Burley 2000). While genetics as a discipline distances itself from eugenics, it remains a reductionist project, albeit with diagnosis as its clinical focus (Kerr and Cunningham-Burley 2000).

The potential to detect genetic predispositions for disease, for example, may lead to many discriminatory practices reminiscent of eugenic "selective breeding" and "racial hygiene." This is notable in insurance coverage, where genetic testing, as well as (one presumes) technologies yet to come, provides a new range of risk profiles that insurers are loath to assume, incorporating premodern notions of fatalism (Kerr and Cunningham-Burley 2000).

Prenatal diagnosis is another area where technology is playing an increasingly wide role. From amniocentesis to chorionic villus sampling and nuchal translucency, tests provide input on the genotype and potential abnormalities. Regardless of the discourse surrounding the testing, be it reassurance that the baby is going to be normal or control over what types of babies a woman can have, the pragmatic outcome of prenatal diagnosis is generally geared toward selective abortion and the elimination of fetuses with genetic defects (Lippman 1991). I am not here expressing a judgment about selective abortion but underlining the fact that the outcome of diagnostic technology, in this case, emphasizes medical rather than social diagnosis and intervention. This raises the question, for example, Is Down syndrome (one prevalent prenatal diagnostic object) an undesirable condition or simply a variant of the range of ways of being? The stigmatization of the individual with Down syndrome focuses on perceived negative potentials (present in all unborn, unraised children, whose intellectual capacities are neither known nor fixed) rather than on other aspects of individual personality.

Privileging certain traits through technologies of prenatal selection presents a new eugenics, putatively based on neoliberal, individual choice rather than governmental coercion or force. However, it has been suggested that there is an implicit coercion, emerging from medical authority and discriminatory beliefs about disability (Raz 2009). Being a carrier of a genetic marker for a particular diagnosis may result in discriminatory practices. Screening programs, such as the Dor Yeshorim premarital genetic testing for potential spouses in ultraorthodox Jewish communities, result in the reinforcement of stigma of those who are presumed to be genetic carriers (Raz and Vizner 2009).

Kerr and Cunningham-Burley (2000) maintain that genetic testing reflects modernist claims about knowledge and control. The technologies may yet be superficial and uncertain, but they are approached, for a variety of reasons, with a certainty and an imperative toward action: "Risk estimates become definitive diagnoses which form part of a chain of diagnostic procedures, starting with counseling and proceeding to abortion, prophylactic treatment or further monitoring" (p. 289).

Hope

Technology cannot be viewed simply as a tool of social control, ensuring patient compliance and reinforcing the hegemonic "medical-industrial complex with dark motives and dependent victims" (Timmermans and Berg 2003, p. 98), playing a game of biological or genetic selection. Technology is not constructed in a vacuum; it is infiltrated and shaped by medical beliefs, professional priorities, lay and social anxieties. In addition to classifying, discriminating, and screening, technology also clearly buttresses therapeutic directions.

Timmermans and Berg posit that sociology has much to offer technology when disciplinary boundaries are put to one side and insights about autonomy, patienthood, and embodied experience can be presented to technology designers. While, on the one hand, I have discussed the potential for technology to trump embodied experience and for technological findings to dominate the clinical hermeneutic, we can equally invest great hope in the potential that technology may offer.

Tragically, Suzanne Fleischmann (1999), whose reflections on the language of disease I have cited regularly throughout this book, died a young woman. Her essay—part personal documentary, part exercise in medical semantics, as she described it—drew on her experience of a rare (and ultimately fatal) illness. In it, technology was paradoxically both the signatory to her death warrant and a vector of hope. "My dreams would conjure up kaleidoscopic images of chromosomes, gene products, transcription factors, and Freudian fragments of damaged DNA longing for repair. Perhaps one of those dreams will engineer a technology for fixing chromosomal breaks in hematopoietic stem cells" (p. 5), she wrote wistfully.

The technology of diagnosis has many potentials. It can emancipate and oppress, clarify and obfuscate, or legitimize medical attitudes and identities (Wailoo 1997, p. 45). For Fleischmann, and indeed for anyone who has endured the transformative insult of the malignant diagnosis, technology is an important life raft. Each test and each therapeutic undertaking raises hope in the remote possibility that an explanation (or even better, a solution) will issue from the next new finding. This may in part explain the American fascination, described by L. M. Schwartz and colleagues (2004), with technological profiles, however imprecise. They are like the pill I imagined as a little girl, the one that science would certainly discover for me, that would let me live forever. Science is always ever just on the brink of solving our problems, I believed, among which mortality is probably the highest priority.

Hope also emerges in the technologies of chronic illness, where instrumental understandings of the body contribute to self-awareness and identity. For example, women who had bone scans to detect osteoporosis wanted these images, whatever stories they told. They felt the images revealed an inner truth about themselves that was not otherwise accessible. This fostered new understandings about themselves and their body image. In this case, the bone scan provided a view of the body object in ways that reorganized their body space and gave different meanings to their experiences of embodiment (Reventlow, Hvas, and Malterud 2006).

Genetic technology enables women with *BRCA1* and *BRCA2* mutations to identify their marked increased risk of breast and ovarian cancer. Women who have these mutations can choose to have both breasts removed even in the absence of any sign of disease. One cohort study over six years showed a reduction in breast cancer of 95 percent in those who elected for double mastectomy (Rebbeck et al. 2004). The decision to opt for mastectomy is nonetheless a difficult choice. Not all women who are *BRCA1* or *BRCA2* positive will have cancer, although the risk is high.

An important theme in syndromes such as the medically unexplained symptom and chronic fatigue is the hope that technology will be able to transform suffering into a legitimized medical condition rather than an elusive and invisible state of maladaption. When the laboratory test or the radiographic image concur with the phenomenological experience of illness, the individual has access to a biomedical explanation, which in turn provides social recognition of his or her suffering (Hydén and Sachs 1998). One important function served by diagnostic testing is visual revelation; that which is neither visually inscribed on the body (it doesn't "show") nor previously validated by medicine gains substance through its inscription in visual imaging (Rhodes et al. 1999). The CT provides, as one informant explained, "solid proof. It [isn't] just aches and pains anymore" (Rhodes et al. 1999, p. 1194). What the patient had "been saying to her doctor could not be heard until, to her joy, it could be seen" (Rhodes et al. 1999, p. 1195). This position of hope reverberates with the case I presented of my own cough. Being able to "see" the illness in its scientized existence would have made my condition real and treatable, as opposed to the unfortunate dilemma it had become within an objectified, diagnostically organized medicine.

Hope is fueled not only by technology's potential to cure but also by its status as a commodity in the free market. Consumer longing for eternal good health and belief in science as an objective yet beneficent purveyor of worthwhile technologies is a practical marketing object within commodity culture. Archie Alexander (2007) describes the United States as the "land of medical imaging opportunity, where anyone can participate in the ultrasound imaging experience" (p. 1). Technology systems can be purchased, and technology experiences can be marketed outside of medical prescription. The ultrasound about which Alexander writes goes beyond its usual diagnostic use to become the plaything of the rich consumer. Tom Cruise, we understand, purchased his own ultrasound machine in order to "visit" his gestating son whenever the mood struck him.

I have elsewhere described how the previously acquiescent patient has received access to information formerly restricted to medicine as a result of new media. This e-scaping[3] is complemented by the increasing presence of diagnostic technologies as consumer products, available outside of medical networks. "Fetal Keepsake Imaging," for example, offers expectant parents a prenatal view of their infant, albeit without a qualified imager to report results, provide standard counseling, or diagnostic examinations (Alexander 2007). The current ambiguity around the appropriate regulations to apply to nonmedical use of this technology (no longer diagnostic but commemorative) creates the mechanisms and incentives for biotechnology companies to market directly to the consumer (as well as to the entrepreneur), with little concern for possible morbidities associated with screening, or alternatively, with the false reassurance about undetected anomalies.

The place of technology in medicine is immense, and the little glimpse contained in these few thousand words barely scratches the surface of its impact in diagnosis. I have not, for example, explored the role of technology in lay and professional education and communication. Nor have I discussed the fuzzy line between genetic enhancement and genetic manipulation that technology offers. What once might have been considered a disadvantage might, in the presence of the ability to "fix" it, become a disease, or a condition worthy of repair, perhaps on the basis that it creates an inferiority complex (see Gilman's 1991 discussion of the "Jewish nose" as an example). I have not even touched on the economics of diagnostic technology. Economic considerations feature in the design and use of diagnostic tests and of the treatments that ensue (Laking, Lord, and Fischer 2006).

Technology is not freely allocated, but it produces dramatic differences in ethnic, demographic, and national diagnostic trends. What we are capable of diagnosing depends not only on our technological ability to diagnose but also on the availability of the equipment to access the technology. In developing countries, in remote and rural areas, and in underprivileged neighborhoods, diagnostic tools taken for granted elsewhere are inaccessible. Even simple biomechanical injuries might never be diagnosed in nations such as the Cook Islands or Tokelau, where x-ray is the only imaging technology available. A CT or an MRI might be as far as three days away by slow boat.

The story of technology's contribution to diagnosis within a social and cultural frame does not end with this chapter. It is a story that is yet to be told, given the ever-changing nature of technologies available for diagnostic purposes. It is, however, a story that can be generically recognized as we study the sociology of diagnosis, because it is an important framing device in diagnostic categories and concordant therapeutic reactions.

Conclusion

Directions for the Sociology of Diagnosis

> People who suffer from compassion fatigue often have high and unrealistic ideas about how they can help others. They believe they should be able to give endlessly, heal everyone and always be right. . . . This can also lead to frustration or anger in workplaces such as hospitals or rest homes where there is a high level of fatigue or stress . . . certain personalities are also more vulnerable to compassion fatigue.   VENITIA SHERSON (2010)

The term *compassion fatigue* was first mooted in the nursing literature in the late 1980s. A Spanish nursing journal published a warning about its existence: "Contact with disease and death, with the suffering of the others . . . demands great psychological stability and creates tremendous stress in those professionals that live day to day with their patients" (La fatiga de la compasión 1989, p. 9), the journal's editor wrote, pleading with nurses to seek help and support. Following in its wake, publications in the fields of medicine and other caring professions started speaking about compassion fatigue. They focused on the exhaustion and psychological distress that resulted from the burden of caring for others who suffer (Booth 1991; Cassidy 1991; Joinson 1992). This burnout, or psychological exhaustion, was cast as a disorder. Joinson (1992) described the symptoms of compassion fatigue to nurses: "You forget or lose things or have a shorter attention span. You're exhausted and have frequent headaches or stomachaches. Your resistance is low and you get sick more often. You're depressed. One particular sign to watch for is anger, especially when it's too frequent and too intense for the situation" (p. 119).

There is growing interest in the strains experienced by those who care (emotionally and physically) for others who suffer. This is perhaps more noticeable as financial and political imperatives restructure the ways in which care is provided. The management of mental illness, disability, special needs, and palliative care is increasingly shrugged off by institutional or state providers, without compensatory development of support structures for the communities and individuals who take on the responsibility. Families are more dispersed, providing only frail networks of mutual assistance.

The newspaper article from which the epigraph is drawn vividly describes the empathy required to be a nurse, the emotional strain of looking after exceptionally ill people day after day with little help or recognition. That the challenges of this often draining, sometimes rewarding, but always demanding devotion to others should be described in the idiom of disease is a commanding reminder of how diagnosis infuses the ways in which we make sense of our difficulties in Western society. *Compassion fatigue, secondary victimization, compassion contagion, burnout syndrome, countertransference,* and *secondary traumatic stress disorder* are all used to describe the burden of caring (Sabo 2006). Compassion fatigue is referred to as a "condition," with victims, symptoms, screening tools, risk factors, and treatments. It has awareness projects, advocates, and perhaps one day will have its very own drugs.

Classifying compassion fatigue as a disorder powerfully demonstrates how disease categories reflect society's anxieties and frame social reality. The notion of "disorder" positions a particular experience (in this case, distress) as pathological or diseased (Horwitz 2007; Horwitz and Wakefield 2007). *Disorder* conveys a different meaning than *distress*. Distress is the unhappy reaction that an individual might experience when faced with a significant social affront—say, the death of a loved one, the loss of a job, or ill health. With distress, the reaction comes from the external condition, or the social affront. As time goes on and the context improves, the individual should recover equilibrium, albeit not necessarily without sequelae or scars. Distress, one might say, is the normal reaction to an abnormal situation: how one would expect to feel when facing something intensely difficult. A disorder, on the other hand, is an abnormal response. It can be a reaction to either a normal or an abnormal situation. That is to say, it can be an overreaction to something that should normally not cause distress, or it can be disordered distress that exceeds the range of typical reactions to the particular situation. A disordered reaction is linked to an internal psychological dysfunction and is located in the individual rather than in the social affront (Horwitz 2007).

Adams et al.'s (2006) study provides a helpful example of how compassion fatigue has been cast as disorder. This study focuses on assessing a screening implement and its predictive validity in compassion fatigue. To do so, the researchers undertook a cross-sectional survey of social workers, chosen because of the high case loads and low resourcing that characterize the field. Despite using a definition of *compassion fatigue* that describes it as "the *natural* consequent behaviors and emotions resulting from knowing about a traumatizing event experienced or suffered by a person" (p. 103, emphasis added)—a definition in line with the idea of stress rather than disorder—the study looks closely at characteristics of the *individual* to explain the cause. The authors consider what aspects of the health care provider's personal history and coping ability might explain or predict the development of compassion fatigue, looking at correlations between general health, stress, and psychological resources, and the putative disorder. This situates the locus of the condition in the individual, shifting it from normal response to disorder.

Far from wishing to deny that those who bear heavy emotional burdens in order to care for others may suffer from their load, I would like nonetheless to propose alternative models for considering compassion fatigue. As mentioned above, Adams and colleagues focus on a dysfunction situated in the individual, trying to detect a frailty or predisposing factor for compassion fatigue. The authors see this work as a "prelude to devising intervention strategies designed to mitigate the negative effects on the care-giving practitioner" (p. 108). The screening tool focuses firmly on the individual and opens the door for interventions within a disease model.

An economic or political framing of this problem would not deny its existence but would situate its cause and remedy outside of the individual, in structural and political action. Had a labor rather than a psychiatric researcher decided to take on this study, she or he might have more intuitively chosen to look at workload and resourcing to understand in what circumstances one is more likely to feel distressed by helping traumatized or suffering individuals. Looking at compassion fatigue as the dysfunction of the individual rather than as a failure of the system closes off a number of other avenues for succor. Social policy and legislation may go further than individual treatment to eradicate what is probably not as prevalent a "disorder" as it is cast to be but is probably an even bigger "problem."

But this is not terribly surprising. That the burden of compassion should be portrayed in terms of disease may also be a strategic mechanism by which the challenge can be better understood. Didier Fassin has spoken of how diagnoses bear witness to the world in authoritative ways. A diagnosis of PTSD brings credibility to subjective accounts of misery from those who have suffered natural disaster, war, or a combination of both. The diagnosis substitutes the words of the expert for the voice of the sufferer (Fassin 2009). In this sense diagnosis mediates suffering and translates it into terms that can no longer be ignored by national and international communities. The DSM-like, technocratic language of medicine compels action as it appropriates and transforms a narrative of human suffering to one of public health imperative.

The example of suffering depicted as disease underlines and epitomizes the social intrigue of diagnosis with which this book is concerned. Diagnosis tells us much about what we value and believe in as people; it behooves us to understand it well. Turner's (2007) and Shermis's (1962) work on new disciplines recommends that to anchor a field, one must consider and define what that field is and how it adds value to society's goals and aspirations. In response to these criteria, a sociology of diagnosis must be concerned with the creation, application, allocation, and exploitation of diagnostic categories.

Creation

What counts as disease and how is this determined? Seeking to understand the classification of diseases and disease discovery processes is a rich source of study. Disease boundaries are ever-shifting, as they negotiate where and how deviance becomes disease, feeling becomes symptom, and the stigmatized becomes value free (Rosenberg 2006, p. 407). The development of diagnoses serves as an indication of what we are prepared to accept as normal, healthy, moral, and bearable. As new disease categories are recognized and incorporated into medicine's taxonomies, they draw together competing and concordant forces: lay activism can both buttress and dispute medical diagnosis.

Technology shifts diagnostic boundaries, just as education, resources, and social priorities shape technology's directions. Technology sees what is invisible to the naked eye. Elevated C-reactive protein, sickling cells, calcifications, and microfibrillary tangles indicate what sicknesses we can have. The human genome project, for example, ultimately proposes a different way of classifying, relying on genetic susceptibility, until now unconsidered in the ICD and DSM.

Application

I have struggled throughout this text to find the mot juste to express the transfer of the diagnosis from the medical lexicon and the doctor's understanding of disease to the lay person's experience of illness. When the patient goes to the doctor, it is to await a kind of stamp, or signet. Its mark determines what happens next, as the condition finds its expression in words that have meaning beyond the individual's perception. The experience of discomfort gets filed with the panoply of other experiences, which together make sense to a wider world. The lay person "gets diagnosed," a passive reidentification over which she or he has less control than one might like, and during which the person's illness becomes validated (or not). This is Blaxter's "process" of diagnosis (Blaxter 1978). Is a diagnosis conveyed? (No, too passive, too much like a property transaction.) Awarded? (Possibly, when having the label opens doors.) Branded (when it's a stigmatizing diagnosis)? Applied (like trying on new lipstick)? Or disclosed (when the severity and complexity of the condition requires a particular discretion and authority)?

Diagnosis is relational and strongly influenced by the positions occupied by doctor and lay person—sometimes on opposing, sometimes on supporting sides. Anatole Broyard (1995) writes of his experience of diagnosis: "Just as he orders blood tests and bone scans of my body, I'd like my doctor to scan *me*, to grope for my spirit as well as my prostate. While he inevitably feels superior to me because he is the doctor and I am the patient, I'd like him to know that I feel superior to him too, that he is my patient also and I have my diagnosis of him. There should be a place where our respective superiorities could meet and frolic together" (p. 179).

The changing roles that are played by lay and professional give pause. Freedom and autonomy, reliance and compliance, all parry and circle around the diagnosis and its application, conveyance, award, branding, or stamp.

Allocation

The diagnosis-resource link has threaded through this book, as it threads through the Western experience of disease. Parson's (1958) early work on the sick role makes clear the first important resource: allowance. The diagnosis entitles the sick person to a different social expectation: the patient rests, misses work, gets help. It is the patient's due.

While I have cited both Freidson and de Swaan in reference to the power imbued in medicine, which serves as the gatekeeper of resources, I will reprise their arguments here with a focus on diagnosis. They both knew that diagnosis was key in the allocation process. Recall that Freidson (1970) wrote, "Where illness is the ubiquitous label for deviance in an age, the profession that is custodian of the label is ascendant" (p. 244). De Swaan (1989) focused on how, in the presence of scant resources, doctors were called on to make decisions about the distribution of goods such as housing, leave, insurance coverage, and treatment. Custodianship of the diagnostic label is shifting, as we can see from the changing nature of the lay-professional relationship, the mediatization of health, and the free flow of previously restricted-access medical information. But the diagnosis remains at the fulcrum of allocation.

Consider, for example, the authorization of particular medications, notably expensive ones. In many cases it is not enough for the doctor simply to diagnose and prescribe. Adalimumab is a case in point. Adalimumab is a monoclonal antibody that reduces the symptoms of ankylosing spondylitis, an inflammatory disease, mainly affecting the spine, with often serious impact on the daily function of those who have it (McLeod et al. 2007). However, given the high cost of this treatment, it is not given without formal diagnostic confirmation of serious ankylosing spondylitis. In New Zealand, for example, access to treatment by Adalimumab is authorized only after a checklist of diagnostic criteria is submitted to the pharmaceutical management agency. The presence of sacroiliitis on x-rays and certain elevated nonspecific clinical markers (ESR and CRP) are prerequisites to treatment (Pharmac 2010). In this case and others like it, the doctor has a role in diagnosis but is powerless to override the administrative definition of the disease, whose standardized criteria fulfill the gatekeeping role. This speaks to what Turner describes as "the standardization of illness into phenomena which can be managed by bureaucratic agencies" (qtd. in Filc 2006).

Exploitation

Diagnoses provide fodder for exploitation: commercial, political, and personal. The "mongering" of diseases (Payer 1992) is not restricted to Big Pharma. The manufacturers of medical equipment, complementary and alternative therapies, nutritional supplements, and food products equally have an interest in promoting particular disease states. Television and media reap benefit from disease stories. Reality television features the fight against obesity (*The Biggest Loser, Weighing In, Celebrity Fit Club*); documentaries highlight personal battles against illness and disease education; self-help books, magazines, and infomercials often have disease as their focus. Gyms and fitness centers generate memberships on the basis of collective concern about obesity, hypertension, and other forms of cardiovascular disease.

An individual might exploit diseases, using the (false) pretext of a headache or influenza to miss work. Being sick is an acceptable reason for not going to work, whereas "getting the car registered before I get a ticket" is not. Taken to an extreme, malingering is the more severe exploitation of diagnostic status by an individual for personal benefit. *Malingering* implies fabricating symptoms in order to receive a diagnosis for some form of secondary gain. Not only might a malingerer shirk work or other social responsibilities, he or she might also pursue financial entitlements, medications, allowances, or simply attention that would otherwise not be permitted.

The fact that diagnoses can be exploited doesn't mean that any one diagnosis is more or less worthy than another, more or less "real." Rather, it reflects the power that putting a name to a condition generates. The fixed disease entity provides substance around which support and interest can rally and a range of agendas be met.

Moving Forward

I have been playing with Ockham's razor myself as I put this book together. I have attempted to look for patterns and boundaries in the study of disease, demonstrating what ideas might cogently be put together, what forces and effects are linked to one another, distinct from others and like enough to make sense to readers when placed in the same chapter. This process of classifying is the means by which we all make social sense of the world, making labels (words) that we can then use among ourselves to communication our interests, hopes, and fears.

The important point, as Nick Fox and Katie Ward (2008) write, is that there is nothing prior and independent about health and disease. Rather, they are assemblages both borne of and acting to reconfirm relations and effects. Health and illness are political categories, they write, resulting just as much from "the physical and cultural possibilities and constraints *surrounding* a person's body as with any characteristic of the body itself" (p. 1019, emphasis added).

A model for a sociology of diagnosis would inevitably need to consider disease as more than a given, a priori entity. This does not mean presuming that diagnostic categories are somehow neither real nor useful. Rather, it means considering how and why particular diseases are framed as they are and not in another way. It implies understanding the interest directed at some conditions as opposed to others and the desirability of some disease labels as contrasted with the unattractiveness of others.

The model depicted in figure 1 recognizes the assemblage that constitutes diagnosis, the relational nature of the diagnostic moment, and the transformative potential of diagnosis as process. I do not propose the fragments that constitute the social framing and social consequences of diagnosis as absolute or complete categories. Reality is continuous, and deciding to lump or to split on the basis of an argument that I propose to my peers is a social action (Zerubavel 1996). It is convention, the same as that "which transforms actual oceans into mental archipelagos" (p. 427). I have in this spirit created categories into which I am forcing reality with the fervor of the foregoing pages to convince my readers that my concept formation is sound.

The model in figure 1 summarizes my thinking but also is a challenge to the discipline for considering whether these pieces fit together and, if not, how they should be modified to do so. A conversation on this subject is important to the field; as an emerging intellectual discipline, the sociology of diagnosis must have "techniques suitable for dealing with its concepts in order to develop a sustainable intellectual tradition" (Shermis 1962, p. 84) and, by extension, contribute to society's goals and aspirations (Turner 2007).

Figure 1 illustrates a consideration of how classifications are generated. Many forces and agents interact to create diagnoses and their consequences. However, these factors are not independent, in their own genesis, from their social consequence: it is a kind of chicken-and-egg situation. While diagnoses cannot import a social consequence until they become standardized as a label, the impact of the label continues to feed into the framing of diagnostic categories as they are, or as they will become. With each revision of the *Diagnostic and Statistical Manual of Mental Disorders* or of the *International Statistical Classification of Diseases*, there are drawn-out debates about how changing a diagnostic category will affect the treatment of disease or the experience of those labeled with disease or about how current categories either achieve or

SOCIAL FRAMING

SOCIAL CONSEQUENCE

| CLASSIFICATION SYSTEMS (historical and contemporary) | DISEASE DISCOVERY | | ALLOCATION | EXPLOITATION |
| RISK PROFILES AND SURVEILLANCE | DIAGNOSTIC TECHNOLOGIES | MD–LAY Interaction | LEGITIMIZATION | STIGMATIZATION |

Figure 1. Social understanding of diagnosis

fail to fulfill their promise. We have explored how lay movements, as well as commercial exploitation, have fed into the social framing of diagnostic categories. In the case of homosexuality, stigmatization drove the movement to change its diagnostic status. On the other hand, the drive for recognition of female hypoactive sexual desire disorder is largely driven by pharmaceutical industry interests.

But this is not a one-way model. Just as the social consequences of diagnosis mold the disease classifications, so do the classifications frame the experiences of diagnosis, a point that hardly needs amplification. As one example, state employees of Alabama have been compelled since 2009 to subject themselves to an annual medical examination including the measurement of BMI. Those who are subsequently diagnosed as obese face an increased insurance premium (Fernandez 2008). This diagnosis results in the immediate consequence of financial penalty. In contrast, diagnosis and impairment ratings are at the heart of disability determination in the case of fibromyalgia and other illnesses that result in work incapacity (Hadler 1996). An individual seeking disability payments would see the diagnosis as key in their pursuit.

In both of these cases, the consequences of the diagnosis (stigmatization for the obese and resources for those with fibromyalgia) feed into the circular relationship described above. Patient advocacy groups, researchers, and insurers will all have their ideas about how better to frame the problems of chronic fatigue or obesity.

The dynamic social nature of diagnosis and the diagnostic process is an important point of academic reflection precisely because diagnoses are not prior, ontological entities but social categories that organize, direct, explain, and sometimes control our experience of health and illness. Bowker and Star (1999) describe classifications as a kind of "work practice," but an invisible one, valorizing some points of view and silencing others (p. 50). The inevitable privileging of certain voices over others in medical classification is opaque and must be made visible. The model proposed above for the sociological analysis of diagnosis provides a tool for revealing the points of view that are contained in a disease label.

The power of sociological analysis is its potential to reveal the deep layers of negotiation, compromise, and interests that cover and surround the scientific evidence of a disease. The assemblages and boundaries that circumscribe disease often have an untapped elasticity that social inquiry can both challenge and reconfigure.

Notes

Introduction

1. This concern was not new. Thomas Percival discussed it in his 1803 *Medical Ethics*: "Falsehood may lose the essence of lying, and become even praiseworthy," he wrote, "when the adherence to truth is incompatible with the practice of some other virtue of still higher obligation" (Percival 1985, p. 160).

CHAPTER TWO: Social Framing and Diagnosis

1. By referring to *baby*, I would confer, wittingly, personhood to the prenatal entity that may or may not ultimately be born. Alternatively, I could refer to the *fetus*, which would suggest a nonautonomous being. Either solution is problematic in a discussion that revolves around the implications contained in language.

2. The term *miscarriage* simultaneously acknowledges and denies fetal personhood. On one hand, it distinguishes the child from the womb: an object to be transported, delivered, and potentially dropped. On the other, the statutory and cultural practices that accompany a miscarriage remove the autonomy of personhood upon the ending of the pregnancy, as I will discuss later. The child becomes a fetus, which is denied the trappings of death.

3. Here, the medical sense of early death, rather than criminal procurement, is implied by the word *abortion*.

4. One obesity action group in New Zealand uses the acronym FOE, or "Fight the Obesity Epidemic."

CHAPTER THREE: What's Wrong with Me?

1. The adjective *patient* is used consciously, with an awareness of the overlapping significance of its nominal and adjectival forms.

CHAPTER FOUR: Beyond Our Ken?

1. Full details of the review summarized here can be found in Jutel 2010b.

2. This approach may be paradoxical, but it is not surprising. Medicine has had a variety of historical mechanisms for arranging that which does not fit into current nosology, from reflex theory to spinal irritation, hysteria, dissociation, and others (Shorter 1992).

3. A number of publications explore the histories of particular diseases, many of which are useful for punctuating the contexts in which these diseases emerged and gained purchase, including, among others, Aronowitz 1998; Packard et al. 2004; Horwitz and Wakefield 2007; Rosenberg and Golden 1992; and others.

CHAPTER FIVE: Driving Diagnosis

1. See Shifren et al. 2008.

2. See Clayton et al. 2009.

3. See Sills et al. 2005.

4. The controversy remains unresolved in that the tentative diagnosis of LLPDD was placed in a special appendix titled "Proposed Diagnostic Categories Needing Further Study" within the DSM-III-R. In the DSM-IV, LLPDD has been renamed "premenstrual dysphoric disorder" and is still located in the appendix as a disputed disorder requiring further study (Busfield and Campling 1996).

5. Since this book went to press, Boehringer Ingelheim made application to the FDA for the approval of flibanserin for the treatment of hypoactive sexual desire disorder (HSDD) in premenopausal women. However, the reproductive drugs panel voted 11–0 that the drug's dubious benefits did not outweigh its side effects. Approval was not granted. Subsequently, Boehringer Ingelheim announced that they would discontinue the development of the compound, maintaining nonetheless that flibanserin provided what they believed was a positive benefit-risk ratio for women living with HSDD. "The need for a better understanding of HSDD and its possible treatment continues," said Michael Sand, Director, Clinical Research and Global Strategic Leader for flibanserin, "and we hope the scientific and medical communities will build on the knowledge that Boehringer Ingelheim's research has provided to find potential treatment options for women who live with this condition" (Boehringer Ingelheim press release, Ridgefield, CT, October 8, 2010). This statement further underlines the role that the pharmaceutical industry plays in promoting diagnostic awareness.

CHAPTER SIX: "There Is Nothing So Small as to Escape Our Inquiry"

1. The social consequences of this discovery included profound racial prejudices and beliefs about "negro blood" and the necessity of segregation to protect the white race (see Wailoo 1997).

2. While Robert Koch, building on the work of René Laennec, provided us with the foundation for the modern definition and conceptualization of tuberculosis, evidence of tuberculosis-like disease is found in ancient archeological remains in Egypt, in classical Greek texts (when it was known as phthisis), in Hippocratic writings, in the biblical books of Deuteronomy and Leviticus, and in ancient India, China, and the Americas (Daniel 2006).

3. See Nettleton 2004.

References

Aalton, C. M., M. M. Samson, and P. A. F. Jansen. 2006. Diagnostic errors: The need to have autopsies. *Netherlands Journal of Medicine* 64 (6):186–90.

Abenhaim, Lucien, Michel Rossignol, Jean-Pierre Valat, Margareta Nordin, Bernard Avouac, Francis Blotman, Jacques Charlot, Renee Liliane Dreiser, Erick Legrand, Sylvie Rozenberg, and Philippe Vautravers. 2000. The role of activity in the therapeutic management of back pain: Report of the International Paris Task Force on Back Pain. *Spine* 24 (4S):1–33S.

Abraham, John. 2007. Building on sociological understandings of the pharmaceutical industry or reinventing the wheel? Response to Joan Busfield, Pills, power, people. *Sociology* 41 (4):727–36.

Alexander, Archie. 2007. "Just scanning around" with diagnostic medical ultrasound: Should states regulate the non-diagnostic use of this technology? *Annals of Health Law* 16 (1):1–42.

Amaducci, Luigi. A., Walter. A. Rocca, and Bruce S. Schoenberg. 1986. Origin of the distinction between Alzheimer's disease and senile dementia: How history can clarify nosology. *Neurology* 36 (11):1497–99.

American Psychiatric Association. 1980. *Diagnostic and Statistical Manual of Mental Disorders* (3d. ed.). Washington, DC: American Psychiatric Association.

———. 1987. *Diagnostic and Statistical Manual of Mental Disorders* (3d. ed., text revisions). Washington, DC: American Psychiatric Association.

———. 2000. Generalized anxiety disorder. In *Diagnostic and Statistical Manual* (4th ed., text revisions). Washington, DC: American Psychiatric Association.

Anon. 1840. *Petites études de la nature ou entretiens recréatifs d'une mère avec ses deux filles sur l'histoire naturelle des animaux et des plantes; les phénomenes astronomiques, et les progrès des arts, des sciences et de la civilisation.* Paris: Niogret.

Anon. 1886. The nomenclature of medicine. *British Medical Journal* 1 (1328):1114–28.

Apple, Rima D. 1995. Constructing mothers: Scientific motherhood in the nineteenth and twentieth centuries. *Social History of Medicine* 8 (2):161–78.

Armstrong, David. 1995. The rise of surveillance medicine. *Sociology of Health and Illness* 17 (3):393–404.

Arnold, Thomas. 1839. *On the Divisions and Mutual Relations of Knowledge: A Lecture Read before the Rugby Literary and Scientific Society, April 7, 1835.* Rugby, UK: Combe and Crossley.

Arnow, Bruce A., Enid Hunkeler, Christine Blasey, Janelle Lee, Michael Constantino, Bruce Fireman, Helena Kraemer, Robin Dea, Rebecca Robinson, and Chris Hayward. 2006. Comorbid depression, chronic pain, and disability in primary care. *Psychosomatic Medicine* 68 (2):262–68.

Aronowitz, Robert. 1998. *Making Sense of Illness: Science, Society, and Disease*. Cambridge: Cambridge University Press.

———. 2001. When do symptoms become a disease? *Annals of Internal Medicine* 134 (9 part 2):803–8.

———. 2008. Framing disease: An underappreciated mechanism for the social patterning of health. *Social Science and Medicine* 67 (1):1–9.

Ayer's Sarsaparilla. 1896. Beauty begins in the blood. *Godey's*, January, 115.

Augustine. 1990. *Sermons II*. Translated by E. Hill. New York: New City Press.

Balint, Michael. 1964. *The Doctor, His Patient and the Illness* (2d ed.). Kent, UK: Pitman Medical.

Ban, Thomas. A. 2006. The role of serendipity in drug discovery. *Dialogues in Clinical Neuroscience* 8 (3):335–44.

Barker, Kristin K. 1998. A ship upon a stormy sea: The medicalization of pregnancy. *Social Science and Medicine* 47 (8):1067–76.

Barsky, Arthur J., and Jonathan F. Borus. 1999. Functional somatic syndromes. *Annals of Internal Medicine* 130 (11):910–21.

Basson, Rosemary, Jennifer Berman, Arthur Burnett, Leonard Derogatis, David Ferguson, Jean Fourcroy, Irwin Goldstein, Allesandra Graziottin, Julia Heiman, Ellen Laan, Sandra Leiblum, Harin Padma-Nathan, Raymond Rosen, Kathleen Segraves, R. Taylor Segraves, Ridwan Shabsigh, Marcalee Sipski, Gorm Wagner, and Beverly Whipple. 2000. Report of the International Consensus Development Conference on Female Sexual Dysfunction: Definitions and classifications. *Journal of Urology* 163 (3):888–93.

Becker, Gay, and Robert D. Nachtigall. 1992. Eager for medicalisation: The social production of infertility as a disease. *Sociology of Health and Illness* 14 (4):456–71.

Berger, Peter L., and Thomas Luckmann. 1966. *The Social Construction of Reality: A Treatise in the Sociology of Knowledge*. Garden City, NY: Doubleday.

Berlin, Leonard, and Jonathan W. Berlin. 2005. Leasing imaging facilities to referring physicians: Fee shifting or fee splitting? *Radiology* 234 (1):44–48.

Bertillon, Jacques. 1909. *Nomenclatures des maladies: Statistique de morbidité—Statistique des causes de décès*. Paris: Montevrain.

Best, Joel. 1989. Afterword. In *Images of Issues: Typifying Contemporary Social Problems*, edited by J. Best. New York: Aldine deGruyter.

Black, William C. 2000. Overdiagnosis: An underrecognized cause of confusion and Harm in cancer screening. *Journal of the National Cancer Institute* 92 (16):1280–82.

Blaxter, Mildred. 1978. Diagnosis as category and process: The case of alcoholism. *Social Science and Medicine* 12:9–17.

———. 2009. The case of the vanishing patient? Image and experience. *Sociology of Health and Illness* 31 (5):762–78.

Boehringer Ingelheim GmbH. 2008. Hypoactive sexual desire disorder backgrounder. *Boehringer Ingelheim Science and Technology Communications*, May.

Bogaert, Anthony F. 2004. Asexuality: Prevalence and associated factors in a national probability sample. *Journal of Sex Research* 41 (3):279–87.

Bonnie, Richard J. 2002. Political abuse of psychiatry in the Soviet Union and in China: Complexities and controversies. *Journal of the American Academy of Psychiatry and the Law* 30:136–44.

Booth, Eric W. 1991. Compassion fatigue. *Journal of the American Medical Association* 266 (3):362.

Borsini, Franco, and Kenneth. R. Evans. 2006. Method of treating female hypoactive sexual desire disorder with Flibanserin. U.S. Patent 7151103 (10/272603).

Borsini, F., E. Giraldo, E. Monferini, G. Antonini, M. Parenti, G. Bietti, and A. Donetti. 1995. BIMT-17, a 5-HT2A receptor antagonist and 5-HT1A receptor full agonist in rat cerebral cortex. *Naunyn-Schmiedebergs Archives of Pharmacology* 352 (3):276–82.

Borsini, F., R. Cesana, J. Kelly, B. E. Leonard, M. McNamara, J. Richards, and L. Seiden. 1997. BIMT-17: A putative antidepressant with a fast onset of action? *Psychopharmacology* 134 (4):378–86.

Bove, A. A. 2008. Internet-based medical education. *Perspectives in Biology and Medicine* 51 (1):61–70.

Bowker, Geoffrey C. 1996. The history of information infrastructures: The case of the international classification of diseases. *Information Processing and Management* 32 (1):49–61.

Bowker, Geoffrey C., and Susan Leigh Star. 1999. *Sorting Things Out: Classification and Its Consequences*. Cambridge, MA: MIT Press.

———. 2000. Invisible mediators of action: Classification and the ubiquity of standards. *Mind, Culture, and Activity* 7 (1):147–63.

Brady, Anita. 2007. *Constituting Queer: Performativity and Commodity Culture, Media Studies*. PhD diss., University of Otago, Dunedin.

Bricart, Isabelle. 1985. *Saintes ou pouliches: L'éducation des jeunes filles au XIXème siècle*. Paris: Albion Michel.

Brody, Howard. 2006. Informed refusal. *Virtual Mentor* 8 (1):24–29.

Brown, David Allen, et al. 2001. *Virtue and Beauty: Leonardo's Ginevra de' Benci and Renaissance Portraits of Women*. Princeton, NJ: Princeton University Press.

Brown, Phil. 1990. The name game: Toward a sociology of diagnosis. *Journal of Mind and Behaviour* 11 (3–4):385–406.

———. 1995. Naming and framing: the social construction of diagnosis and illness. *Journal of Health and Social Behavior* Health Module:34–52.

———. 2008. Naming and framing: The social construction of diagnosis and illness. In *Perspectives in Medical Sociology*, edited by P. Brown. Long Grove, IL: Waveland Press.

Brown, Phil, and Stephen Zavestoski. 2004. Social movements in health: An introduction. *Sociology of Health and Illness* 26 (6):679–94.

Brown, Phil, Stephen Zavestoski, Sabrina McCormick, Brian Mayer, Rachel Morello-Frosch, and Rebecca Gasior Altman. 2004. Embodied health movements: New approaches to social movements in health. *Sociology of Health and Illness* 26 (1): 50–80.

Broyard, Anatole. 1995. Doctor, talk to me. In *On Doctoring*, edited by R. Reynolds and J. Stone. New York: Simon & Schuster.

Buetow, Stephen A. 2005. To care is to coprovide. *Annals of Family Medicine* 3 (6): 553–55.

Buetow, Stephen A., Annemarie Jutel, and Karen Hoare. 2009. Shrinking social space in the doctor–modern patient relationship: A review of forces for, and implications of, homologisation. *Patient Education and Counseling* 74 (1):97–103.

Burgan, Mary. 2005. Superstars and rookies of the year: Faculty hiring practices in the post-modern age. Center for Studies in Higher Education Research and Occasional Papers Series CSHE.10.05:1–17.

Burr, Vivien. 1995. *An Introduction to Social Constructionism.* London: Routledge.

Busfield, Joan. 2006. Pills, power, people: Sociological understandings of the pharmaceutical industry. *Sociology* 40 (2):297–314.

Busfield, Joan, and Jo Campling. 1996. *Men, Women, and Madness: Understanding Gender and Mental Disorder.* Washington Square, NY: New York University Press.

California Fig Syrup Company. 1896. Syrup of Figs. *Godey's*, January, back cover.

Campos, Paul, Abigail Saguy, Paul Ernsberger, Eric Oliver, and Glenn Gaesser. 2006. The epidemiology of overweight and obesity: Public health crisis or moral panic? *International Journal of Epidemiology* 35 (1):55–60.

Carey, John. 2006. Viagra for women? *Businessweek*, 28 December, www.business week.com/bwdaily/dnflash/content/dec2006/db20061228_315249.htm (accessed 19 October 2009).

Cartwright, Samuel A. 1981. Report of the diseases and physical peculiarities of the Negro race. In *Concepts of Health and Disease*, edited by A. Caplan, H. T. Engelhardt, and J. McCartney. Reading, MA: Addison-Wesley Publishing Co.

Carver, Raymond. 1998. What the doctor said. In *All of Us: The Collected Poems.* New York: Knopf.

Cassell, Eric J. 1991. *The Nature of Suffering and the Goals of Medicine.* New York: Oxford University Press.

Cassidy, J. 1991. Compassion fatigue: Healthcare professionals are vulnerable as care giving becomes more stressful. *Health Progress* 72 (1):54–55, 64.

Caux, Chantal, David J. Roy, Louise Guilbert, and Claude Viau. 2007. Anticipating ethical aspects of the use of biomarkers in the workplace: A tool for stakeholders. *Social Science and Medicine* 65 (2):344–54.

Centers for Disease Control and Prevention. 2005. Diseases and conditions. www .cdc.gov/node.do/id/0900f3ec8000e035 (accessed 30 November 2005).

———. 2009. Interim guidance on infection control measures for 2009 H1N1 influenza in healthcare settings, including protection of healthcare personnel.

www.cdc.gov/h1n1flu/guidelines_infection_control.htm (accessed 16 November 2009).

CFIDS Association of America. 2009. Do I have CFS? www.cfids.org/about-cfids/do-i-have-cfids.asp (accessed 20 November 2009).

Charland, Louis C. 2004. A madness for identity: Psychiatric labels, consumer autonomy, and the perils of the Internet. *Philosophy, Psychiatry, and Psychology* 11 (4):336–49.

Christie, William F. 1927. *Surplus Fat and How to Reduce It*. London: Heinemann / Medical Books.

Clark, Jack A., and Elliot G. Mishler. 1992. Attending to patients' stories: Reframing the clinical task. *Sociology of Health and Illness* 14 (3):344–72.

Clarke, Adele E., and Monica J. Casper. 1996. From simple technology to complex arena: Classification of Pap smears, 1917–90. *Medical Anthropology Quarterly* 10 (4):601–23.

Clarke, Adele E., Janet K. Shim, Laura Mamo, Jennifer Ruth Fosket, and Jennifer R. Fishman. 2003. Biomedicalization: Technoscientific transformations of health, Illness, and U.S. biomedicine. *American Sociological Review* 68 (2):161–94.

Clayton, Anita H., Evan R. Goldfischer, Irwin Goldstein, Leonard Derogatis, Diane J. Lewis-D'Agostino, and Robert Pyke. 2009. Validation of the decreased sexual desire screener (DSDS): A brief diagnostic instrument for generalized acquired female hypoactive sexual desire disorder (HSDD). *Journal of Sexual Medicine* 6 (3):730–38.

Cochrane, Archie L. 1989. Archie Cochrane in his own words: Selections arranged from his 1972 introduction to *Effectiveness and Efficiency: Random Reflections on the Health Services* 1972. *Control Clinical Trials* 10 (4):428–33.

Cohen, Marc S. 2008. Aristotle's *Metaphysics*. In *Stanford Encyclopedia of Philosophy*, edited by E. N. Zalta. Stanford, CA: Metaphysics Research Lab. plato.stanford.edu/entries/aristotle-metaphysics/#Cat.

Cohen, Stanley. 1980. *Folk Devils and Moral Panics: The Creation of the Mods and Rockers*. New York: St. Martin's Press.

Conrad, Kathryn. 2001. Foetal Ireland: National Bodies and Political Agency. *Eire-Ireland*, Fall–Winter, 157–73.

Conrad, Peter. 1975. The discovery of hyperkinesis: Notes on the medicalization of deviant behavior. *Social Problems* 23 (1):12–21.

———. 1979. Types of medical social control. *Sociology of Health and Illness* 1 (1):1–11.

———. 1992. Medicalization and social control. *Annual Review of Sociology* 18: 209–32.

———. 2005. The shifting engines of medicalization. *Journal of Health and Social Behavior* 46 (1):3–14.

———. 2007. *The Medicalization of Society: On the Transformation of Human Conditions into Treatable Disorders*. Baltimore: Johns Hopkins University Press.

Conrad, Peter, and Valerie Leiter. 2004. Medicalization, markets and consumers. *Journal of Health and Social Behavior* 45 (Suppl.):158–76.

Conrad, Peter, and Joseph Schneider, W. 1980. *Deviance and Medicalization: From Badness to Sickness.* St. Louis: C. V. Mosby Co.

Corbett, Kevin, and Tristen Westwood. 2005. "Dangerous and severe personality disorder": A psychiatric manifestation of the risk society. *Critical Public Health* 15 (2):121–33.

Cowan, L., and M Wainwright. 2001. The death of a baby in our care: The impact on the midwife. *Midwifery Digest* 11 (3):313–16.

Croskerry, Pat. 2002. Achieving quality in clinical decision making: Cognitive strategies and detection of bias. *Academic Emergency Medicine* 9 (11):1184–1205.

Cushman, Philip. 1990. Why the self is empty: Toward a historically situated psychology. *American Psychologist* 45 (5):599–611.

Daniel, Thomas M. 2006. The history of tuberculosis. *Respiratory Medicine* 100 (11):1862–70.

Deale, Alicia, and Simon Wessely. 2001. Patients' perceptions of medical care in chronic fatigue syndrome. *Social Science and Medicine* 52 (12):1859–64.

Dear, James W., and David J. Webb. 2007. Disease mongering: A challenge for everyone involved in healthcare. *British Journal of Clinical Pharmacology* 64 (2):122–24.

Derogatis, Leonard R., Raymond Rosen, Sandra Leiblum, Arthur Burnett, and Julia Heiman. 2002. The female sexual distress scale (FSDS): Initial validation of a standardized scale for assessment of sexually related personal distress in women. *Journal of Sex and Marital Therapy* 28 (4):317–30.

De Swaan, Abram. 1989. The Reluctant imperialism of the medical profession. *Social Science and Medicine* 28 (11):1165–70.

Dewhurst, Kenneth. 1966. *Dr. Thomas Sydenham, 1624–1689: His Life and Original Writings.* Berkeley: University of California Press.

Dietary Guidelines Advisory Committee. 1995. *Report of the Dietary Guidelines Advisory Committee on the Dietary Guidelines for Americans.* Washington, DC: U.S. Department of Agriculture.

Dixon, Jane, and Cathy Banwell. 2004. Re-embedding trust: Unravelling the construction of modern diets. *Critical Public Health* 14 (2):117–31.

Dumit, Joseph. 2006. Illnesses you have to fight to get: Facts as forces in uncertain, emergent illnesses. *Social Science and Medicine* 62 (3):577–90.

Durham, John. 2002. Population screening for prostate cancer: A systematic review. In *New Zealand Guidelines Group.* Wellington, NZ: University of Otago Department of General Practice.

Durkheim, Emile, and Marcel Mauss. 1903. De quelques formes de classification: Contribution à l'étude des représentations collectives. *Année Sociologique* 6:1–72.

Emanuel, Ezekiel J., and Linda L. Emanuel. 1992. Four models of the physician-patient relationship. *Journal of the American Medical Association* 267 (16):2221–26.

Engelhardt, H. Tristram. 1992. The body as a field of meaning: Implications for the ethics of diagnosis. In *The Ethics of Diagnosis*, edited by J. L. Peset and D. Gracia. Dordecht, Netherlands: Kluwer Academic Publishers.

Epstein, Steven. 1996. *Impure Science: AIDS, Activism, and the Politics of Knowledge.* Berkeley: University of California Press.

Erlbeck, Hana H. 2001. *The Legends of the Demi-God Maui-Tikitiki-a-Taranga.* Auckland, NZ: Reed.

Evidence-Based Medicine Working Group. 1992. Evidence-based medicine: A new approach to teaching the practice of medicine. *Journal of the American Medical Association* 268 (17):2420–25.

Fassin, Didier. 2009. Global public health. Presentation at Medical Anthropology at the Intersections: Celebrating 50 Years of Interdisciplinarity, Yale University.

Feldman, Simon D., and Alfred I. Tauber. 1997. Sickle cell anemia: Reexamining the first "molecular disease." *Bulletin of the History of Medicine* 71 (4):623–50.

Fernandez, Don. 2008. Alabama "obesity penalty" stirs debate. CBS News Health, August 25. www.cbsnews.com/stories/2008/08/25/health/webmd/main4382340 .shtml.

Ferris, D. G., C. Dekle, and M. S. Litaker. 1996. Women's use of over-the-counter antifungal medications for gynecologic symptoms. *Journal of Family Practice* 42 (6):595–600.

Ferris, D. G., P. Nyirjesy, J. D. Sobel, D. Soper, A. Pavletic, and M. S. Litaker. 2002. Over-the-counter antifungal drug misuse associated with patient-diagnosed vulvovaginal candidiasis. *Obstetrics and Gynecology* 99 (3):419–25.

Filc, Dani. 2006. Power in the primary care medical encounter: Domination, resistance and alliances. *Social Theory and Health* 4:221–43.

Fischer-Homberger, Esther. 1970. Eighteenth-century nosology and its survivors. *Medical History* 14 (4):397–403.

Flegal, Katherine M. 2006. Commentary: The epidemic of obesity: What's in a name? *International Journal of Epidemiology* 35 (1):72–74, discussion on 81–82.

Flegal, Katherine M., Barry I. Graubard, David. F. Williamson, and Mitchell H. Gail. 2005. Excess deaths associated with underweight, overweight, and obesity. *Journal of the American Medical Association* 293 (15):1861–67.

Fleischman, Suzanne 1999. I am . . . , I have . . . , I suffer from . . . : A Linguist reflects on the language of illness and disease. *Journal of Medical Humanities* 20 (1):1–31.

Fleiss, Joseph L., William Lawlor, Stanley R. Platman, and Ronald R. Fieve. 1971. On the use of inverted factor analysis for generating typologies. *Journal of Abnormal Psychology* 77 (2):127–32.

Foucar, Elliot 2001. Classification in anatomic pathology. *American Journal of Clinical Pathology* 116 (Suppl.):S5–S20.

Foucault, Michel. 1963. *Naissance de la clinique.* Paris: Presses Universitaires de France.

Fox, Nick, and Katie Ward. 2006. Health identities: From expert patient to resisting consumer. *Health* (London) 10 (4):461–79.

———. 2008. What are health identities and how may we study them? *Sociology of Health and Illness* 30 (7):1007–21.

Fox, Nick, Katie Ward, and Alan O'Rourke. 2005. Pro-anorexia, weight-loss drugs and the Internet: An "anti-recovery" explanatory model of anorexia. *Sociology of Health and Illness* 27 (7):944–71.

Fox, Patrick. 1989. From senility to Alzheimer's disease: The rise of the Alzheimer's disease movement. *Milbank Quarterly* 67 (1):58–102.

Frances, A. 2010. Opening Pandora's box: The 19 worst suggestions for DSM-5. *Psychiatric Times*, www.psychiatrictimes.com/dsm/content/article/10168/1522341.

Frank, Arthur W. 1995. *The Wounded Storyteller: Body, Illness, and Ethics.* Chicago: University of Chicago Press.

Freemantle, Nick, and Mel Calvert. 2007. Composite and surrogate outcomes in randomised controlled trials. *British Medical Journal* (334):756–57.

Freidson, Eliot. 1970. *Profession of Medicine: A Study of the Sociology of Applied Knowledge.* New York: Dodd, Mead & Co.

Furedi, Frank. 2006. The end of professional dominance. *Society* 43 (6):14–18.

Gaesser, Glenn A. 1999. Has body weight become an unhealthy obsession? *Medicine and Science in Sports and Exercise* 31:1118–28.

Gaines, Atwood D. 1992. From DSM-I to III-R; voices of self, mastery and the other: A cultural constructivist reading of U.S. psychiatric classification. *Social Science and Medicine* 35 (1):3–24.

Galdas, Paul M., Francine Cheater, and Paul Marshall. 2005. Men and help-seeking behaviour: Literature review. *Journal of Advanced Nursing* 6:616–23.

Gallo, Robert C., and Luc Montagnier. 2003. The discovery of HIV as the cause of AIDS. *New England Journal of Medicine* 349 (24):2283–85.

Getz, Linn, Johann A. Sigurdsson, Irene Hetlevik, Anna L. Kirkengen, Solfrid Romundstad, and Jostein Holmen. 2005. Estimating the high risk group for cardiovascular disease in the Norwegian HUNT 2 population according to the 2003 European guidelines: Modelling study. *British Medical Journal* 331 (7516):551.

Gevitz, Norman. 2000. "The Devil hath laughed at the physicians": Witchcraft and medical practice in seventeenth-century New England. *Journal of the History of Medicine* 55 (1):5–36.

Gilman, Sander L. 1991. *The Jew's Body.* New York: Routledge.

Goldstein, Annemarie. 2007. Medicine's flight from interpretation: When a cough is simply a cough. *Clinical Ethics* 2 (1):15–18.

Goldstein, Dianne E. 2004. Communities of suffering and the Internet. In *Emerging Illnesses and Society: Negotiating the Public Health Agenda,* edited by R. M. Packard, P. J. Brown, R. L. Berkelman and H. Frumkin. Baltimore: Johns Hopkins University Press.

Goode, Erich. 1969. Marijuana and the politics of reality. *Journal of Health and Social Behavior* 10 (2):83–94.

Graber, Mark, Ruthanna Gordon, and Nancy Franklin. 2002. Reducing diagnostic errors in medicine: What's the goal? *Academic Medicine* 77 (10):981–92.

Graunt, John. 1662. *Natural and Political Observations, Mentionned in a following Index, and made upon the Bills of Mortality.* London: John Martin, James Allestry, and the Dicas.

Grimes, David A., and Kenneth F. Schulz. 2005. Surrogate end points in clinical research: Hazardous to your health. *Obstetrics and Gynecology* 105 (5 [part 1]):1114–18.

Gurwitz, Jerry H., Thomas J. McLaughlin, and Leslie S. Fish. 1995. The effect of an Rx-to-OTC switch on medication prescribing patterns and utilization of physician services: The case of vaginal antifungal products. *Health Services Research* 30 (5):672–85.

Hacking, Ian. 2001. Inaugural lecture: Chair of philosophy and history of scientific concepts at the Collège de France, 16 January 2001. *Economy and Society* 31 (1):1–14.

Hadler, Norman M. 1996. If you have to prove you are ill, you can't get well: The object lesson of fibromyalgia. *Spine* 21 (20):2397–2400.

Han, Paul K. 1997. Historical changes in the objectives of the periodic health examination. *Annals of Internal Medicine* 127 (10):910–17.

Harrington, Patricia, and Marvin D. Shepherd. 2002. Analysis of the movement of prescription drugs to over-the-counter status. *Journal of Managed Care Pharmacy* 8 (6):499–508, quiz on 509–11.

Hayes, Brett, and Roger Adams. 2008. Parallels between clinical reasoning and categorization. In *Clinical Reasoning in the Health Professions*, edited by J. Higgs, S. Loftus, and N. Christensens. Oxford: Butterworth-Heinemann.

Health Funding Authority. 1999. New Zealand mothers and babies: An analysis of national maternity data. Hamilton, NZ: Health Funding Authority.

Healy, David. 2006. The latest mania: Selling bipolar disorder. *PLoS Medicine* 3 (4):e185.

Hebl, Mikki R., and J. Xu. 2001. Weighing the care: Physicians' reactions to the size of a patient. *International Journal of Obesity and Related Metabolic Disorders* 25 (8):1246–52.

Henwood, Flis, Sally Wyatt, Angie Hart, and Julie Smith. 2003. "Ignorance is bliss sometimes": Constraints on the emergence of the "informed patient" in the changing landscapes of health information. *Sociology of Health and Illness* 25 (6):589–607.

Herrick, S. S. 1889. *A Reference Handbook of the Medical Sciences.* Edited by A. H. Buck. Edinburgh: Pentland.

Herxheimer, Andrew. 2003. Relationships between the pharmaceutical industry and patients' organisations. *British Medical Journal* 326:1208–10.

Hesse, Bradford W., David E. Nelson, Gary L. Kreps, Robert T. Croyle, Neeraj K. Arora, Barbara K. Rimer, and Kasisomayajula Viswanath. 2005. Trust and sources of health information: The impact of the Internet and its implications for health care providers; findings from the first Health Information National Trends Survey. *Archives of Internal Medicine* 165 (22):2618–24.

Hippocrates. 1983. Prognosis. In *Hippocratic Writings*, edited by G. E. R. Lloyd. London: Penguin.

Hollick, Frederick. 1902. *The Origin of Life and Process of Reproduction in Plants and Animals, With the Anatomy and Physiology of the Human Generative System, Male and Female, and the Causes, Prevention and Cure of the Special Diseases to Which It Is Liable: A Plain, Practical Treatise, for Popular Use.* Philadelphia: David McKay.

Horwitz, Allan V. 2007. Distinguishing distress from disorder as psychological outcomes of stressful social arrangements. *Health* (London) 11 (3):273–89.

Horwitz, Allan V., and Jerome C. Wakefield. 2007. *The Loss of Sadness: How Psychiatry Transformed Normal Sorrow into Depressive Disorder.* New York: Oxford University Press.

Houlihan, Catherine F., Sanjay Patel, David. A. Price, Manoj Valappil, and Uli Schwab. 2010. Life threatening infections labelled swine flu. *British Medical Journal* 340:c137.

Hunter, Kathryn Montgomery. 1991. *Doctors' Stories: The Narrative Structure of Medical Knowledge.* Princeton, NJ: Princeton University Press.

Hydén, Lars-Christer, and Lisbeth Sachs. 1998. Suffering, hope and diagnosis: On the negotiation of chronic fatigue syndrome. *Health* (London) 2 (2):175–93.

Illich, Ivan. 1976. *Limits to Medicine: Medical Nemesis, the Expropriation of Health.* Middlesex, UK: Penguin.

Jackson, Mark. 1996. "Something more than blood": Conflicting accounts of pregnancy loss in eighteenth-century England. In *The Anthropology of Pregnancy Loss: Comparative Studies in Miscarriage, Stillbirth and Neonatal Death*, edited by R. Cecil. Oxford: Berg.

Jackson, Stanley W. 1978. Melancholia and the waning of the humoral theory. *Journal of the History of Medicine and Allied Sciences* 33 (3):367–76.

Jacob, Elin K. 1992. Classification and categorization: drawing the line. *Advances in Classification Research: Proceedings of the ASIS SIG/CR Classification Research Workshop* 2:67–83.

Jagose, Annamarie. 2003. Against love. Paper delivered to the Department of Cinema Studies, New York University, New York, NY, 7 February.

Jepson, Ruth. 2006. Informed refusal. *Virtual Mentor* 8 (1):24–29.

Jerome, Jerome K. 1889. *Three Men in a Boat (To Say Nothing of the Dog).* London: J. W. Arrowsmith.

Joinson, C. 1992. Coping with compassion fatigue. *Nursing* 22 (4):116, 118–19, 120.

Jutel, Annemarie. 2001. Does size really matter? Weight and values in public health. *Perspectives in Biology and Medicine* 44 (2):283–96.

———. 2005. Weighing health: The moral burden of obesity. *Social Semiotics* 15 (2):113–25.

———. 2006a. The emergence of overweight as a disease entity: Measuring up normality. *Social Science and Medicine* 63 (9):2268–76.

———. 2006b. What's in a Name? Death before birth. *Perspectives in Biology and Medicine* 49 (3):425–34.

———. 2007. Medicine's flight from interpretation: When a cough is simply a cough. *Clinical Ethics* 2(1): 15–18.

———. 2008. Doctor's orders: Diagnosis, medicalisation and the exploitation of anti-fat stigma. In *Biopolitics and the "Obesity Epidemic": Governing Bodies*, edited by J. Wright and V. Harwood. New York: Taylor & Francis.

———. 2010a. Framing disease: The example of female hypoactive sexual desire disorder. *Social Science and Medicine* 70:1084–90.

——— 2010b. Medically unexplained symptoms and the disease label. *Social Theory and Health* 8:229–45.

Jutel, Annemarie, and Stephen A. Buetow. 2007. A picture of health? Unmasking the role of appearance in health. *Perspectives in Biology and Medicine* 50 (3):421–34.

Kahn, Eugen. 1957. The life and work of Emil Kraepelin. *Association of Schools of Public Health* 72 (7):527–74.

Kaplan, H. S. 1977. Hypoactive sexual desire. *Journal of Sex and Marital Therapy* 3 (1):3–9.

Kastelein, J. J., F. Akdim, E. S. Stroes, A. H. Zwinderman, M. L. Bots, A. F. Stalenhoef, F. L. Visseren, E. J. Sijbrands, M. D. Trip, E. A. Stein, D. Gaudet, R. Duivenvoorden, E. P. Veltri, A. D. Marais, and E. de Groot. 2008. Simvastatin with or without ezetimibe in familial hypercholesterolemia. *New England Journal of Medicine* 358 (14):1431–43.

Kerr, Anne, and Sarah Cunningham-Burley. 2000. On ambivalence and risk: Reflexive modernity and the new human genetics. *Sociology* 34 (2):283–304.

Kilbourne, Jean. 2003. Advertising and disconnection. In *Sex in Advertising*, edited by T. Reichert and J. Lambiase. Mahwah, NJ: Lawrence Erlbaum Associates.

Kipen, H. M., and N. Fiedler. 2002. Environmental factors in medically unexplained symptoms and related syndromes: The evidence and the challenge. *Environmental Health Perspectives* 110 (Suppl. 4):597–99.

Kirk, Stuart A., and Herb Kutchins. 1992. *The Selling of DSM: The Rhetoric of Science in Psychiatry.* New York: Aldine de Gruyter.

Kirmayer, Laurence J., Danielle Groleau, Karl J. Looper, and Melissa D. Dao. 2004. Explaining medically unexplained symptoms. *Canadian Journal of Psychiatry* 49 (10):663–71.

Klawiter, Maren. 1999. Racing for the cure, walking women, and toxic touring: Mapping cultures of action within the Bay Area terrain of breast cancer. *Social Problems* 46 (1):104–26.

———. 2004. Breast cancer in two regimes: The impact of social movements on illness experience. *Sociology of Health and Illness* 26 (6):845–74.

Kleinman, Arthur. 1988. *The Illness Narratives: Suffering, Healing, and the Human Condition.* New York: Basic Books.

Kleinman, Arthur, Leon Eisenberg, and Byron Good. 1978. Culture, illness, and care: Clinical lessons from anthropologic and cross-cultural research. *Annals of Internal Medicine* 88 (2):251–58.

Klinkenborg, Verlyn. 1994. Dangerous diagnoses. *New Yorker*, July 18, 78–80.

Kolker, Emily S. 2004. Framing as a cultural resource in health social movements: Funding activism and the breast cancer movement in the U.S., 1990–1993. *Sociology of Health and Illness* 26 (6):820–44.

Kuczmarski, Robert J., and Katherine M. Flegal. 2000. Criteria for definition of overweight in transition: Background and recommendations for the United States. *American Journal of Clinical Nutrition* 72 (5):1074–81.

Kutchins, Herb, and Stuart A. Kirk. 1989. DSM-III-R: The conflict over new psychiatric diagnoses. *Health and Social Work* 14 (2):91–101.

———. 1997. *Making Us Crazy : DSM: The Psychiatric Bible and the Creation of Mental Disorders.* New York: Free Press.

La fatiga de la compasión. Editorial. 1989. *Revista de Enfermeria* 12 (136):9.

Laking, George, Joanne Lord, and Alastair Fischer. 2006. The economics of diagnosis. *Health Economics* 15 (10):1109–20.

Lancet. 1897. Notes, short comments and answers to correspondents: The reliance personal weighing machine, May 8, 1316.

Laqueur, Thomas. 1990. *Making Sex: Body and Gender from the Greeks to Freud.* Cambridge, MA: Harvard University Press.

Lavater, John Caspar. 1855. *Essays on Physiognomy—Designed to Promote Knowledge and Harmony among Mankind* (15th ed.). Translated by T. Holcroft. London: William Tegg.

Lawn, J. E., M. Y. Yakoob, R. A. Haws, T. Soomro, G. L. Darmstadt, and Z. A. Bhutta. 2009. 3.2 million stillbirths: Epidemiology and overview of the evidence review. *BMC Pregnancy Childbirth* 9 (Suppl. 1):S2.

Leder, Drew. 1990. Clinical interpretation: The hermeneutics of medicine. *Theoretical Medicine* 11:9–24.

Lee, Shirley, and Avis Mysyk. 2004. The medicalization of compulsive buying. *Social Science and Medicine* 58 (9):1709–18.

Lemon, George William. 1701. *English Etymology; or a Derivative Dictionary of the English Language in Two Alphabets.* London: G. Robinson.

Leray, Jean. 1931. *Embonpoint et obésité: Conceptions et thérapeutiques actuelles.* Paris: Massion et Cie.

Lexchin, Joel. 2006. Bigger and better: How Pfizer redefined erectile dysfunction. *PLoS Medicine* 3 (4):1–4.

Lief, Harold I. 1977. Inhibited sexual desire. *Medical Aspects of Human Sexuality* 7: 94–95.

Light, Donald, and Sol Levine. 1988. The changing character of the medical profession: A theoretical overview. *Milbank Quarterly* 66:10–32.

Lippman, Abby. 1991. Prenatal genetic testing and screening: Constructing needs and reinforcing inequities. *American Journal of Law and Medicine* 17 (1&2):15–50.

Locker, David. 1981. *Symptoms and Illness: The Cognitive Organization of Disorder.* London: Tavistock Publications.

Lombroso, Caesar, and William Ferrero. 1895. *The Female Offender.* London: T. Fisher Unwin.

Lorber, Judith, and Lisa Jean Moore. 2002. *Gender and the Social Construction of Illness.* Walnut Creek, CA: Alta Mira Press.

Lunbeck, Elizabeth. 1987. "A new generation of women": Progressive psychiatrists and the hypersexual female. *Feminist Studies* 13 (3):513–43.

Lupton, Deborah. 1997a. Consumerism, reflexivity and the medical encounter. *Social Science and Medicine* 45 (3):373–81.

———. 1997b. Doctors on the medical profession. *Sociology of Health and Illness* 19 (4):480–97.

McEwan, Ian. 2004. The diagnosis. *New Yorker,* 20 December, 116–29.

Madden, Richard, Catherine Sykes, and Bedirhan Ustun. 2007. *World Health Organization Family of International Classifications: Definition, Scope and Purpose.* Geneva: WHO.

Malterud, Kirsti. 1999. The (gendered) construction of diagnosis interpretation of medical signs in women patients. *Theoretical Medicine and Bioethics* 20 (3):275–86.

———. 2000. Symptoms as a source of medical knowledge: Understanding medically unexplained disorders in women. *Family Medicine* 32 (9):603–11.

———. 2001. The art and science of clinical knowledge: Evidence beyond measures and numbers. *Lancet* 358 (9279):397–400.

———. 2005. Humiliation instead of care? *Lancet* 9488:785–86.

Malterud, Kirsti, and A. Taksdal. 2007. Shared spaces of reflection: Approaching the medically unexplained disorder. *Junctures: The Journal for Thematic Dialogue* (9):27–38.

Malterud, Kirsti, Lucy Candid, and Lorraine Code. 2004. Responsible and responsive knowing in medical diagnosis: The medical gaze revisited. *NORA: Nordic Journal of Feminist and Gender Research* 12 (1):8–19.

Marcus, P. M., E. J. Bergstralh, M. H. Zweig, A. Harris, K. P. Offord, and R. S. Fontana. 2006. Extended lung cancer incidence follow-up in the Mayo Lung Project and overdiagnosis. *Journal of the National Cancer Institute* 98 (11):748–56.

Mayes, Rick, and Allen V. Horwitz. 2005. DSM-III and the revolution in the classification of mental illness. *Journal of the History of the Behavioral Sciences* 41 (3):249–67.

McEntee, Michael. 2003. Health screenings: A tool for today's marketers. *Medical Marketing and Media* 38 (2):52–59.

McKinlay, Eileen. 2005. Men and health: A literature review. Wellington, NZ: Department of General Practice, Wellington School of Medicine and Health Sciences, Otago.

McLeod, C., A. Bagust, A. Boland, P. Dagenais, R. Dickson, Y. Dundar, R. A. Hill, A. Jones, R. Mujica Mota, and T. Walley. 2007. Adalimumab, etanercept and infliximab for the treatment of ankylosing spondylitis: A systematic review and economic evaluation. *Health Technology Assessment* 11 (28):1–158.

Meador, Clifton. 2005. *Symptoms of Unknown Origin: A Medical Odyssey.* Nashville: Vanderbilt University Press.

Melechi, Antonio. 2003. *Fugitive Minds: On Madness, Sleep and Other Twilight Afflictions*. London: Arrow Books.

Melendy, Mary Ries. 1904. *Vivilore: The Pathway to Mental and Physical Perfection*. Wellington, NZ: Milton Porter.

Mendelson, George. 2003. Homosexuality and psychiatric nosology. *Australian and New Zealand Journal of Psychiatry* 37 (6):678–83.

Meyer-Kleinmann, Julia. 2008a. Largest study of its kind reveals low sexual desire is most common female sexual problem. *Boehringer Ingelheim Science and Technology Communications*, 31 October.

———. 2008b. Women suffering from decreased sexual desire: Silence hinders diagnosis of the prevalent condition hypoactive sexual desire disorder (HSDD). *Boehringer Ingelheim Science and Technology Communications*, 7 May.

Miller, Fiona A., Megan E. Begbie, Mita Giacomini, Catherine Ahern, and Erin A. Harvey. 2006. Redefining disease? The nosologic implications of molecular genetic knowledge. *Perspectives in Biology and Medicine* 49 (1):99–114.

Miller, Genevieve. 1962. "Airs, waters, and places" in history. *Journal of the History of Medicine and Allied Sciences* 17 (1):129–40.

Milliken, Donald. 1998. Death by restraint. *Canadian Medical Association Journal* 158 (12):1611–12.

Mills, Wilfred. 1977. Definition of perinatal mortality. *Lancet* 25 June:1358.

Ministry of Social Development. 2003. *Unofficial Consolidation of the Social Security Act 1964*. Wellington, NZ: Work and Income New Zealand.

Mintzes, Barbara, Morris L. Barer, Richard L. Kravitz, Arminee Kazanjian, Ken Bassett, Joel Lexchin, Robert G. Evans, Richard Pan, and Stephen A. Marion. 2002. Influence of direct to consumer pharmaceutical advertising and patients' requests on prescribing decisions: Two site cross sectional survey. *British Medical Journal* 324 (7332):278–79.

Mirowsky, John, and Catherine E. Ross. 1989. Psychiatric diagnosis as reified measurement. *Journal of Health and Social Behavior* 30 (1):11–25, discussion on 26–40.

Moncrieff, Joanna, Steve Hopker, and Philip Thomas. 2005. Psychiatry and the pharmaceutical industry: Who pays the piper? *Psychiatric Bulletin* 29:84–85.

Monistat. 2009. Understanding your body. www.monistat.com/understanding-your-body.jsp (accessed 19 November 2009).

Morse, Janice M. 2006. The politics of evidence. *Qualitative Health Research* 16 (3):395–404.

Moynihan, Ray. 2003. The making of a disease: Female sexual dysfunction. *British Medical Journal* 326 (7379):45–47.

Moynihan, Ray, and Alan Cassels. 2005. *Selling Sickness: How Drug Companies Are Turning Us All into Patients*. Sydney: Allen & Unwin.

Moynihan, Ray, Iona Heath, and David Henry. 2002. Selling sickness: The pharmaceutical industry and disease mongering. *British Medical Journal* 324 (7342):886–91.

Mullen, Patricia D. 1997. Compliance becomes concordance. *British Medical Journal* 314 (7082):691–92.

Munro, Robin J. 2002. Political psychiatry in post-Mao China and its origins in the cultural revolution. *Journal of the American Academy of Psychiatry and the Law* 30 (1):97–106.

Murray, T. Jock. 2005. *Multiple Sclerosis: The History of a Disease*. New York: Demos Medical Publishing.

Napheys, George H. 1871. *The Physical Life of Woman: Advice to the Maiden, Wife and Mother* (6th ed.). Philadelphia: George Maclean.

Nettleton, Sarah. 2004. The emergence of e-scaped medicine. *Sociology* 38 (4):661–79.

———. 2006. "I just want permission to be ill": Towards a sociology of medically unexplained symptoms. *Social Science and Medicine* 62 (5):1167–78.

Nettleton, Sarah, Lisa O'Malley, Ian Watt, and Philip Duffey. 2004. Enigmatic illness: Narratives of patients who live with medically unexplained symptoms. *Social Theory and Health* 2:47–66.

Neuberger, Julia. 1999. Do we need a new word for patients? Let's do away with "patients." *British Medical Journal* 318:1756–57.

Nevill, Alan M., Arthur D. Stewart, Tim Olds, and Roger Holder. 2006. Relationship between adiposity and body size reveals limitations of BMI. *American Journal of Physical Anthropology* 129:151–56.

"New inventions." 1899. *Lancet*, 940.

New Zealand College of Midwives. 2004. *Midwifery Standards Review Handbook*. Christchurch, NZ: New Zealand College of Midwives.

Nilsson, P. M., J. A. Nilsson, B. Hedblad, G. Berglund, and F. Lindgarde. 2002. The enigma of increased non-cancer mortality after weight loss in healthy men who are overweight or obese. *Journal of Internal Medicine* 252 (1):70–78.

Novak, Michael. 1965. Toward understanding Aristotle's categories. *Philosophy and Phenomenological Research* 26 (1):117–23.

Ockham, William of. 1997. In *Chambers Biographical Dictionary*, edited by M. Parry. New York: Chambers.

Oliver, J. E. 2006. The politics of pathology: How obesity became an epidemic disease. *Perspectives in Biology and Medicine* 49 (4):611–29.

One News. 2005a. Abandoned baby buried by community. 2 February. tvnz.co.nz/view/news_national_story_skin/471787%3fformat=html.

One News. 2005b. Baby Aaron's mother found. 9 March. tvnz.co.nz/view/news_national_story_skin/478375%3fformat=html.

Orpana, Heather M., Jean-Mari Berthelot, Mark S. Kaplan, David H. Feeny, Bentson McFarland, and Nancy A. Ross. 2009. BMI and mortality: Results from a national longitudinal study of Canadian adults. *Obesity* (Silver Spring) 18 (1):214–18.

Ovid. 1985. *Metamorphoses, Book III*. Translated and edited by D. E. Hill. Warminster, UK: Aris & Phillips.

Pabst Brewing Company. 1897. Pabst Malt Extract. *Godey's*, January, 115.

Packard, R. M., P. J. Brown, R. L. Berkelman, and H. Frumkin (Eds.). 2004. *Emerg-*

ing *Illnesses and Society: Negotiating the Public Health Agenda*. Baltimore: Johns Hopkins University Press.

Paquette, Mary. 2003. Excited delirium: Does it exist? *Perspectives in Psychiatric Care* 39 (3):93–94.

Parry, Vince. 2007. Disease branding: What is it, why it works, and how to do it. *Pharmaceutical Executive*, October, 22–24.

Parsons, Talcott. 1951. Illness and the role of the physician: A sociological perspective. *American Journal of Orthopsychiatry* 21:452–60.

———. 1979. Definitions of health and illness in the light of American values and social structure. In *Patients, Physicians and Illness: Sourcebook in Behavioral Science and Medicine* (3d ed.), edited by E. G. Jaco. New York: Free Press.

Payer, Lynn. 1992. *Disease-Mongers: How Doctors, Drug Companies, and Insurers Are Making You Feel Sick*. New York: John Wiley & Sons.

Percival, Thomas. 1985. *Medical Ethics; or, A Code of Institutes and Precepts, Adapted to the Professional Conduct of Physicians and Surgeons*. Birmingham, AL: The Classics of Medicine Library.

Petchesky, Rosalind P. 1987. Fetal images: The power of visual culture in the politics of reproduction. *Feminist Studies* 13 (2):263–92.

Pharmac. 2010. Application for subsidy by special authority. www.pharmac.govt.nz/2010/04/01/SA0974.pdf (accessed 8 April 2010).

Pilowsky, Issy. 1994. Abnormal illness behaviour: A 25th anniversary review. *Australia New Zealand Journal of Psychiatry* 28:566–73.

Pratt, Lois, Arthur Seligmann, and George Reader. 1958. Physicians' views on the level of medical information among patients. In *Patients, Physicians and Illness: Sourcebook in Behavioral Science and Medicine*, edited by E. G. Jaco. Glencoe, IL: Free Press.

Prause, Nicole, and Cynthia A. Graham. 2007. Asexuality: classification and characterization. *Archives of Sexual Behavior* 36 (3):341–56.

Procter and Gamble. 2009. Beautify your heart. www.metamucil.com/beautify-your-heart/resources-bmi-calculator.php (accessed 30 September 2009).

Procter and Gamble Pharmaceuticals UK, Ltd. 2009. Intrinsa 300 micrograms/24 hours transdermal patch. intrinsa.co.uk/media/downloads/en/Intrinsa%20SPC%2016–09–2008.pdf (accessed 19 October 2009).

Proctor, S. P., T. Heeren, R. F. White, J. Wolfe, M. S. Borgos, J. D. Davis, L. Pepper, R. Clapp, P. B. Sutker, J. J. Vasterling, and D. Ozonoff. 1998. Health status of Persian Gulf War veterans: Self-reported symptoms, environmental exposures and the effect of stress. *International Journal of Epidemiology* 27 (6):1000–1010.

Puhl, R. M., and K. D. Brownell. 2003. Psychosocial origins of obesity stigma: Toward changing a powerful and pervasive bias. *Obesity Reviews* 4:213–27.

Quételet, Adolphe. 1870. *Anthropométrie, ou, Mesure des différentes facultés de l'homme*. Paris: C. Muquardt.

Raz, Aviad E. 2009. Eugenic utopias/dystopias, reprogenetics, and community genetics. *Sociology of Health and Illness* 31 (4):602–16.

Raz, Aviad E., and Yafa Vizner. 2009. Carrier matching and collective socialization in community genetics: Dor Yeshorim and the reinforcement of stigma. *Social Science and Medicine* 67 (9):1361–69.

Reagan, Leslie. J. 2003. From hazard to blessing to tragedy: Representations of miscarriage in twentieth-century America. *Feminist Studies* 13 (2):263–92.

Rebbeck, Timothy R., Tara Friebel, Henry T. Lynch, Susan L. Neuhausen, Laura van 't Veer, Judy E., Garber, Gareth R. Evans, Steven A. Narod, Claudine Isaacs, Ellen Matloff, Mary B. Daly, Olufunmilayo I. Olopade, and Barbara L. Weber. 2004. Bilateral prophylactic mastectomy reduces breast cancer risk in *BRCA1* and *BRCA2* mutation carriers: The PROSE Study Group. *Journal of Clinical Oncology* 22 (6):1055–62.

Reichert, Tom, and Jacqueline Lambiase. 2003. One phenomenon, multiple lenses: Bridging perspectives to examine sex in advertising. In *Sex in Advertising: Perspectives on the Erotic Appeal*, edited by T. Reichert and J. Lambiase. Mahwah, NJ: Lawrence Erlbaum Associates.

Reventlow, Susanne D., Lotte Hvas, and Kirsti Malterud. 2006. Making the invisible body visible: Bone scans, osteoporosis and women's bodily experiences. *Social Science and Medicine* 62 (11):2720–31.

Rhodes, Lorna A., Carol A. McPhillips-Tangum, Christine Markham, and Rebecca Klenk. 1999. The power of the visible: The meaning of diagnostic tests in chronic back pain. *Social Science and Medicine* 48 (9):1189–203.

Richardson, Diane. 2007. Patterned fluidities: (Re)imagining the relationship between gender and sexuality. *Sociology* 41 (3):457–74.

Richardson, Ernest Cushing. 1901. *Classification*. New York: Charles Scribner's Sons.

Roberts, Mary Louise. 1998. Gender, consumption, and commodity culture. *American Historical Review* 103 (3):817–44.

Robins, Lee N., and John E. Helzer. 1986. Diagnosis and clinical assessment: The current state of psychiatric diagnosis. *Annual Review of Psychology* 37:409–32.

Robinson, G. Canby. 1939. *The Patient as Person: A Study of the Social Aspects of Illness*. New York: Commonwealth Fund.

Robinson, K., P. F. Whelan, O. Ghita, and D. Brennan. 2005. Measurement and localization of body fat in whole body MRI. Third Annual IEI Biomedical Engineering Research Award. Dublin.

Rodin, Mari. 1992. The social construction of premenstrual syndrome. *Social Science and Medicine* 35 (1):49–56.

Rogler, Lloyd H. 1997. Making sense of historical changes in the Diagnostic and Statistical Manual of Mental Disorders: Five propositions. *Journal of Health and Social Behavior* 38 (1):9–20.

Romero-Corral, Abel, Victor M. Montori, Virend K. Somers, Josef Korinek, Randal J. Thomas, Thomas G. Allison, Farouk Mookadam, and Francisco Lopez-Jimenez. 2006. Association of bodyweight with total mortality and with cardiovascular events in coronary artery disease: A systematic review of cohort studies. *Lancet* (368):666–78.

Rosecrance, John. 1985. Compulsive gambling and the medicalization of deviance. *Social Problems* 32 (3):275–84.

Rosenberg, Charles E. 1992. *Explaining Epidemics and Other Studies in the History of Medicine*. Cambridge: Cambridge University Press.

———. 2002. The tyranny of diagnosis: Specific entities and individual experience. *Milbank Quarterly* 80 (2):237–60.

———. 2006. Contested boundaries: Psychiatry, disease, and diagnosis. *Perspectives in Biology and Medicine* 49 (3):407–24.

Rosenberg, Charles E., and Janet Golden. (Eds.). 1992. *Framing Disease: Studies in Cultural History*. New Brunswick, NJ: Rutgers University Press.

Rothblum, Esther D., and Kathleen A. Brehony. 1993. *Boston Marriages: Romantic but Asexual Relationships among Contemporary Lesbians*. Amherst: University of Massachusetts Press.

Rothwell, D. J. 1985. Requirements of a national health information system. In *Role of Informatics in Health Data Coding and Classification Systems*, edited by R. A. Cole, D. J. Protti, and J. R. Scherrer. Amsterdam: Elsevier.

Rowley, M. J., M. J. Hensley, M. W. Brinsmead, and J. H. Wlodarczyk. 1995. Continuity of care by a midwife team versus routine care during pregnancy and birth: A randomised trial. *Medical Journal of Australia* 163 (6):289–93.

Russell, Khyla. 2005. Personal communication. Dunedin, NZ.

Ryall, Tony. 2007. Prostate cancer guidelines taking too long. New Zealand National Party press release. www.scoop.co.nz/stories/PA0701/S00063.htm (accessed 7 October 2009).

Sabo, Brenda M. 2006. Compassion fatigue and nursing work: Can we accurately capture the consequences of caring work? *International Journal of Nursing Practice* 12 (3):136–42.

Sarbin, Theodore R., and John I. Kitsuse. 1994. *Constructing the Social: Inquiries in Social Construction*. London: Sage.

Scherrer, Kristin S. 2008. Coming to an asexual identity: Negotiating identity, negotiating desire. *Sexualities* 11 (5):621–41.

Schrader, Catharina. 1987. *"Mother and Child Were Saved": The Memoirs (1693–1740) of the Frisian Midwife Catharina Schrader*. Translated by H. Marland. Amsterdam: Editions Rodophi.

Schwartz, Hillel. 1986. *Never Satisfied: A Cultural History of Diets, Fantasies, and Fat*. New York: Anchor Books.

Schwartz, Lisa M., Steven Woloshin, Floyd J. Fowler Jr., and H. Gilbert Welch. 2004. Enthusiasm for cancer screening in the United States. *Journal of the American Medical Association* 291 (1):71–78.

Scott, Susie. 2006. The medicalisation of shyness: From social misfits to social fitness. *Sociology of Health and Illness* 28 (2):133–53.

Scott, Wilbur, J. 1990. PTSD in DSM-III: A case in the politics of diagnosis and disease. *Social Problems* 37 (3):294–310.

Sharpe, M. 2002. Medically unexplained symptoms and syndromes. *Clinical Medicine* 2 (6):501–4.

Shaykh, Hanan al-. 1994. Inside a Moroccan bath. In *Minding the Body: Women Writers on Body and Soul*, edited by P. Foster. New York: Doubleday.

Sheffield Hearing Voices Network. 2010. Hearing voices network. www.hearingvoices.org (accessed 10 June 2010).

Shermis, Sherwin S. 1962. What makes a subject respectable? On becoming an intellectual discipline. *Phi Delta Kappan* 44 (2):84–86.

Sherson, Venitia. 2010. Caring till it hurts. *Dominion Post*, 13 March, suppl. p. 8–11.

Shifren, Jan L., Brigitta U. Monz, Patricia A. Russo, Anthony Segreti, and Catherine B. Johannes. 2008. Sexual problems and distress in United States women: Prevalence and correlates. *Obstetrics and Gynecology* 112 (5):970–78.

Shorter, Edward. 1992. *From Paralysis to Fatigue: A History of Psychosomatic Illness in the Modern Era*. New York: Free Press.

Sills, Terrence, Glen Wunderlich, Robert Pyke, R. Taylor Segraves, Sandra Leiblum, Anita Clayton, Dan Cotton, and Kenneth Evans. 2005. The Sexual Interest and Desire Inventory–Female (SIDI-F): Item response analyses of data from women diagnosed with hypoactive sexual desire disorder. *Journal of Sexual Medicine* 2 (6):801–18.

Silvestri, L. G., and L. R. Hill. 1964. Some problems of the taxometric approach. In *Phenetic and Phylogenetic Classification*, edited by V. H. Heywood and J. McNeill. London: Systematics Association Publication.

Sim, Julius, and Sue Madden. 2008. Illness experience in fibromyalgia syndrome: A metasynthesis of qualitative studies. *Social Science and Medicine* 67 (1):57–67.

Skegg, Keren. 1993. Multiple sclerosis presenting as a pure psychiatric disorder. *Psychological Medicine* 23 (4):909–14.

Skegg, Keren, P. A. Corwin, and David C. Skegg. 1988. How often is multiple sclerosis mistaken for a psychiatric disorder? *Psychological Medicine* 18 (3):733–36.

Smith-Rosenberg, C., and C. Rosenberg. 1973. The female animal: Medical and biological views of woman and her role in nineteenth-century America. *Journal of American History* 60 (2):332–56.

Sokal, Robert R. 1974. Classification: Purposes, principles, progress, prospects. *Science* 185 (4157):1115–23.

Sontag, Susan. 1978. *Illness as Metaphor*. New York: Farrar, Straus & Giroux.

Sotiriou, Christos, Soek-Ying Neo, Lisa M. McShane, Edward L. Korn, Philip M. Long, Amir Jazaeri, Philippe Martiat, Steve B. Fox, Adrian L. Harris, and Edison T. Liu. 2003. Breast cancer classification and prognosis based on gene expression profiles from a population-based study. *Proceedings of the National Academy of Sciences of the United States of America* 100 (18):10393–98.

Spitzack, Carole. 1990. *Confessing Excess: Women and the Politics of Body Reduction*. Albany: State University of New York Press.

Stafford, Barbara, John La Puma, and David Schiedermayer. 1989. One face of beauty, one picture of health: The hidden aesthetic of medical practice. *Journal of Medicine and Philosophy* 14:213–30.

Star, Susan Leigh, and Geoffrey C. Bowker. 1997. Of lungs and lungers: The classified story of tuberculosis. *Mind, Culture, and Activity* 4 (1):3–23.

Star, Susan Leigh, and James R. Griesemer. 1989. Institutional ecology, "translations" and boundary objects: Amateurs and professionals in Berkeley's Museum of Vertebrate Zoology, 1907–39. *Social Studies of Science* 19 (3):387–420.

Stewart, J. A. 1814. *The Young Woman's Companion; or, Female Instructor: Being a sure and complete guide to every acquirement essential in forming A Pleasing Companion, a Respectable Mother, or A Useful Member of Society.* Oxford: Bartlett and Newman.

Stewart, Jonathan T. 1989. Misdiagnosis of Huntington's disease. *Journal of Neuropsychiatry and Clinical Neurosciences* 1 (1):97.

Stone, Jon, Wojtek Wojcik, Daniel Durrance, Alan Carson, Steff Lewis, Lesley MacKenzie, Charles P. Warlow, and Michael Sharpe. 2002. What should we say to patients with symptoms unexplained by disease? The "number needed to offend." *British Medical Journal* 325 (7378):1449–50.

St-Onge, Myreille, Helene Provencher, and Carl Ouellet. 2005. Entendre des voix: nouvelles voies ouvrant sur la pratique et la recherche. *Santé Mentale au Québec* 30 (1):125–50.

Swayne, Jeremy. 1993. A common language of care? *Journal of Interprofessional Care* 7 (1):29–35.

Sydenham, Thomas. 1742. *The entire works of Dr Thomas Sydenham, newly made English from the originals: . . . To which are added, explanatory and practical notes, from the best medicinal writers. By John Swan, M.D.* London: printed for Edward Cave.

Teachman, B. A., and K. D. Brownell. 2001. Implicit anti-fat bias among health professionals: Is anyone immune? *International Journal of Obesity and Related Metabolic Disorders* 25 (10):1525–32.

Temple, Robert. 1999. Are surrogate markers adequate to assess cardiovascular disease drugs? *Journal of the American Medical Association* 282 (8):790–95.

Thomas, J. 1891. *A Complete Pronouncing Medical Dictionary.* London: Deacon.

Tiefer, Leonore. 1996. The medicalization of sexuality: Conceptual, normative, and professional issues. *Annual Review of Sex Research* 7:252–82.

———. 2006. Female sexual dysfunction: A case study of disease mongering and activist resistance. *PLoS Medicine* 3 (4):e178.

Timmermans, Stefan, and Marc Berg. 2003. The practice of medical technology. *Sociology of Health and Illness* 25 (3):97–114.

Trundle, Catherine. 2010. Commonwealth nuclear test veterans and the quest for recognition. In Graduate School of Nursing, Midwifery and Health Research Seminar Series. Victoria, NZ: University of Wellington.

Turner, Richard C. 2007. Theorizing an emerging discipline: Philanthropic studies. *Nonprofit and Voluntary Sector Quarterly* 36 (4, suppl):163–68S.

Undeland, Merete, and Kirsti Malterud. 2002. Diagnostic work in general practice: More than naming a disease. *Scandinavian Journal of Primary Health Care* 20 (3):145–50.

U.S. Census Bureau. 2004. *Amusement, Gambling, and Recreation Industries, 2002.* Washington, DC: U.S. Census Bureau.

Veith, Ilza. 1981. Historical reflections on the changing concepts of disease. In *Concepts of Health and Disease: Interdisciplinary Perspectives*, edited by A. L. Caplan, H. T. Engelhardt Jr., and J. J. McCartney. Reading, MA: Addison-Wesley Publishing Co.

Vertinsky, Patricia A. 1994. *The Eternally Wounded Woman: Women, Doctors, and Exercise in the Late Nineteenth Century.* Urbana: University of Illinois Press.

Wahab, M. A., E. M. Nickless, R. Najar-M'kacher, C. Parmentier, J. V. Podd, and R. E. Rowland. 2008. Elevated chromosome translocation frequencies in New Zealand nuclear test veterans. *Cytogenetic and Genome Research* 121 (2):79–87.

Wailoo, Keith. 1997. *Drawing Blood: Technology and Disease Identity in Twentieth-Century America.* Baltimore: Johns Hopkins University Press.

Waldenstrom, U., and D. Turnbull. 1998. A systematic review comparing continuity of midwifery care with standard maternity services. *British Journal of Obstetrics and Gynaecology* 105 (11):1160–70.

Ware, Norma C. 1992. Social construction of illness: The delegitimation of illness experience in chronic fatigue syndrome. *Medical Anthropology Quarterly* 6 (4):347–61.

Williamson, Charlotte. 1999. The challenge of lay partnership: It provides a different view of the world. *British Medical Journal* 319 (7212):721–22.

Willis, Thomas. 1681. *The Remaining Medical Works of that Famous and Renowned Physician Dr Thomas Willis.* London: T. Dring, C. Harper, J. Leigh, and S. Martyn.

Wilson, Patricia M. 2001. A policy analysis of the expert patient in the United Kingdom: Self-care as an expression of pastoral power? *Health and Social Care in the Community* 9 (3):134–42.

Winkelman, Warren J., and Chun Wei. Choo. 2003. Provider-sponsored virtual communities for chronic patients: Improving health outcomes through organizational patient-centred knowledge management. *Health Expectations* 6 (4):352–58.

Wolfe, David E. 1961. Sydenham and Locke on the limits of anatomy. *Bulletin of the History of Medicine* 35:193–220.

Wolinsky, Howard. 2005. Disease mongering and drug marketing. *European Molecular Biology Organization Reports* 6 (7):612–14.

Wolters, R., C. Wensing, C. Van Weel, G. J. Van der Wilt, and R. P. T. M. Grol. 2002. Lower urinary tract symptoms: Social influence is more important than symptoms in seeking medical care. *British Journal of Urology International* 90:655–61.

World Health Organization. 1957. *Manual of the International Statistical Classification of Diseases, Injuries and Causes of Death* Geneva: WHO.

———. 1977. *International Statistical Classification of Diseases and Related Health Problems* (9th revision). Geneva: WHO.

———. 1994. *International Statistical Classification of Diseases and Related Health Problems* (10th revision). Geneva: WHO.

———. 2003. *International Statistical Classification of Diseases and Related Health Problems* (10th revision, 2d ed.). Geneva: WHO.

———. 2009a. International classification of diseases (ICD). www.who.int/classifi
cations/icd/en/ (accessed 13 August 2009).

———. 2009b. WHO global infobase. https://apps.who.int/infobase/report.aspx?rid=
114&iso=TON&ind=BMI (accessed 9 September 2009).

Xenical-Orlistat. (2010). Find out your body mass index. www.xenical.com/default
.asp (accessed 28 August 2010).

Yip, Kam-Shing. 2005. An historical review of the mental health services in the People's Republic of China. *International Journal of Social Psychiatry* 51 (2):106–18.

Zavestoski, Stephen, Phil Brown, Meadow Linder, Sabrina McCormick, and Brian Mayer. 2002. Science, policy, activism, and war: Defining the health of Gulf War veterans. *Science, Technology, and Human Values* 27 (2):171–205.

Zerubavel, Eviatar. 1991. *The Fine Line: Making Distinctions in Everyday Life.* New York: Free Press.

———. 1996. Lumping and splitting: Notes on social classification. *Sociological Forum* 11 (3):421–33.

Zola, Irving Kenneth. 1972. Medicine as an institution of social control. *Sociological Review* 20:487–504.

———. 1983. *Socio-Medical Inquiries: Recollections, Reflections, and Reconsiderations.* Philadelphia: Temple University Press.

Index

abortion, xv, 51, 53, 54, 55, 56, 61. *See also* fetal death

ADHD. *See* attention deficit hyperactivity disorder

aesthetics of health, 48

Agent Orange, 90

AIDS, 17

alcoholism, 9

Alzheimer disease, xiii, 92–93, 118

American Psychiatric Association, 31, 34, 113; Committee on Women of, 113

antisocial personality disorder, 80

anti-Soviet thoughts, 80

appearance, 46–48

Aristotle, 19, 37

Armstrong, David, 127–128

Arnold, Thomas, 15, 16

Aronowitz, Robert, 14, 35, 39, 41, 98, 109, 148

asexuality, 105–106. *See also* Boston marriages

attention deficit hyperactivity disorder, 13

authority, medical. *See* medical authority

Balint, Michael, 4, 13, 22, 63

beauty, 47, 48

Bedlam, 31

Bertillon, Jacques, 28

Bertillon Classification, 28

Bethlam. *See* Bedlam

biological markers, 39

black lung, 94

Blaxter, Mildred, xiv, 10, 26, 27, 66, 73, 122, 140

body mass index (BMI), 42–43, 45, 49, 50, 52, 59, 101

Boehringer Ingelheim, 109, 110–112, 114, 115

Boston marriages, 106

Bowker, Geoffrey, 4, 12, 26, 27, 34, 35, 145

BRCA genetic markers, 133

breast cancer, 11, 13, 25, 91, 119, 129, 133

Brown, Phil, 5, 11, 26–27, 31, 41, 68, 72, 76, 79, 88, 89, 91

Carver, Raymond, 62, 75

children's health, 85

chlorosis, 119–120

cholesterol, 128

chronic fatigue syndrome, 41, 71, 78, 83, 90, 105, 133, 145

classification: flexibility of, 16, 143–145; goals of, xiv, 12, 15, 17–23; history of, 6, 21–23; principles of, 4

classification documents and systems: Bertillon Classification, 28; Diagnosis-Related Groups, 29; *Diagnostic and Statistical Manual of Mental Disorders*, 3, 18, 23, 30–4, 80, 88–89, 103, 113, 114, 139, 143; *International Statistical Classification of Diseases and Related Health Problems*, 8, 18, 24, 27–28, 37, 52, 87, 103, 114, 139, 143; Medical Subject Headings, 30; Read Codes, 29; *Statistical Manual for the Use of Institutions of the Insane*, 31; Systemized Nomenclature of Medicine, 29

Clayton, Anita, 4, 108, 109, 111, 112, 115

"clinical hermeneutic," 64

commercial forces, 68, 70, 94, 99, 100, 101. *See also* diet industry; gym industry; pharmaceutical industry

compassion fatigue, 136–139

computed tomography, 126, 133, 135

Conrad, Peter, xvi, 8, 9, 49, 60, 67, 88, 97, 98, 109

consumers, 69, 74, 100, 109–110, 134

contested diagnoses, xvi, 35–36, 77–80, 105

contextual constructionism, 40
Cook Islanders, 37, 50, 135
CT. *See* computed tomography

dangerous and severe personality disorder, 80
da Vinci, Leonardo, 47
decreased sexual desire screener, 108, 115
dementia, xiii
depression, 9, 13, 77, 87, 110, 111, 113, 125, 136
deviance, xiii, 7, 10, 12, 30, 45, 60, 83, 98, 116,
    139, 141
diagnosis: authority to assign, 8; history of, 6
Diagnosis-Related Groups, 29
diagnostic errors, 84
diet industry, 43, 48, 49, 100, 141
direct-to-consumer advertising, 71, 74, 85, 100
disease advocacy, 5, 74, 91, 94, 100
disease discovery, 5, 87–93
disease mongering, 70, 99, 114, 141. *See also*
    pharmaceutical industry
disorder, 137
distress, 137
doctor-patient relationship. *See* patient-doctor
    relationship
Dor Yeshorim, 131
Down syndrome, 131
drapetomania, 3
DSM, 26, 31, 32, 33, 104, 114, 139. *See also*
    under classification documents and systems
DSM-I, 31
DSM-II, 31, 33
DSM-III, 32, 34, 88, 89, 103, 113, 114, 148
DSM-IV, 32, 80, 148
DSM-V, 32
Dumit, Joseph, 35, 77, 78, 79, 88, 95, 105
Durkheim, Emile, 18

Engelhardt, H. Tristram, 21
environmental diseases, 11, 25, 29, 87, 90, 94,
    130
epidemics, 28, 59–60
erectile dysfunction, 122
eugenics, 130, 131
evidence-based practice, 8, 24, 37, 39, 45, 49,
    50, 93, 120, 121
excited delirium, 3, 101
exploitation, 49, 112, 116, 139, 141, 142, 144, 145

Farr, William, 19
Fassin, Didier, 139
female hypoactive sexual desire disorder, 98,
    101, 102–116
fetal death, 51–59
Fetal Keepsake Imaging, 134
fibromyalgia, 77–78, 90, 145
Fleischmann, Suzanne, 2, 132
flibanserin, 110–111, 122, 148
Foucault, Michel, 44, 65, 81, 124
Fox, Nick, 74, 92, 93, 95, 105, 142
France, 2
Frank, Arthur, 65, 66
Freidson, Eliot, 5, 7, 8, 9, 64, 67
funeral grant, 56

Gay Psychiatric Association, 34
genetic discrimination, 130
genetics, xvi, 3, 16, 84, 118, 119, 120–134, 139
gestation, 52, 55, 56, 59
gluttony, 44
Graunt, John, 18, 23, 24, 31
Gulf War–related illness, 90
gym industry, 43, 48, 49, 100, 142

Hacking, Ian, 14, 38
health identities, 74
health outcomes, 55, 66, 86, 95, 128
health social movements, 5, 12, 25, 68, 91, 93,
    95
Hearing Voice Network, 95
hematology, 119, 122
Hippocrates, 42, 62, 69, 113
homosexuality, 3, 17, 32, 33–35, 89, 104
hope, 132–134
Horwitz, Allen, 32, 137, 148
Human Genome Project, 139
humoral theory, 120
Huntington disease, 30
hysteria, 112

identity: collective, 11, 18, 20, 25, 91; health,
    74; individual, xii, 4, 11, 24, 25, 26, 63, 65,
    66, 73, 74, 75, 98, 116, 133; virtual, 11, 95, 105
Illich, Ivan, 12
illness-disease dichotomy, xv, 5, 62, 63, 78,
    84, 96

infanticide, 57
infant mortality, 54
infertility, 4, 9, 21
influenza, 72
insurance coverage, 130
International Statistical Classification of Diseases and Related Health Problems. See under classification documents and systems

Jewish communities, orthodox, 131
"Jewish nose," 134

Kirk, Stuart, 31, 32, 33, 34, 114
Klawiter, Maren, 11, 25
Kleinman, Arthur, 5, 13, 64, 65
Kraepelin, Emil, 92
Kutchins, Herb, 31, 32, 33, 34, 114

late luteal phase dysphoric disorder, 113, 148
Lavater, 43
lay-professional interactions, xv, 13, 76, 81, 93, 140
Leder, Drew, 63, 64, 65, 81, 86, 123, 125
legitimization, xiii, 4, 7, 9, 30, 65, 67, 116, 129, 130, 132, 133, 144
Lemon, George, 6
lesbian, 106
Locke, John, 117
Lombroso, 43
Lupton, Deborah, 8, 67, 93
Lyme disease, 4, 16–17

magnetic resonance imaging, 126, 135
malaria, 72
Malleus Maleficarum, 113
Mary, Virgin, 47
masochistic personality disorder, 114
Mauss, Marcel, 18
Mayes, Rick, 32
medical authority, xiii, 6–10, 67, 68, 69, 72–73, 76, 93
medical dominance. *See* medical authority
medical education, 21–22
medicalization, 5, 9–10, 97–98; and ADHD, 13; of alcoholism, 9; of children's health, 85; of motherhood, 9; of unwanted childless-

ness, 4, 9, 21 (*see also* infertility); of women's health, 85
medically unexplained symptoms, xiii, 11, 35, 80, 82–87
medical power. *See* medical authority
Medical Subject Headings, 30
meningitis, 18
men's health, 85–86
menstruation, 10, 13, 85, 113, 148
microscopy, 117–118
midwifery, 54, 55, 56, 59
migraine, 18
miscarriage, xv, 51, 53, 55, 56. *See also* fetal death
moral panic, 60
Morton foot syndrome, 46
motherhood, 9
MRI, 126, 135
multiple sclerosis, 30, 35

narrative: doctors', 65, 66; patients', 65, 66
Nettleton, Sarah, 8, 65, 69, 79, 84, 93, 100
New Zealand: Baby Aaron, 57–58; Births, Deaths, and Marriage Registration Act, 56, 57; Crimes Act, 55, Māori, 56, 57; politics, 101, 129
Niueans, 50
Norway, 128
nuclear testing, 129

obesity, 42, 43, 46, 59, 61, 100
Ockham's razor, 15, 17, 119, 141
overdiagnosis, 128
over-the-counter medications, 51, 71
overweight, xv, 4, 37–38, 41, 42–51, 60, 121, 145

paresis, 35
Parsons, Talcott, 4, 9, 140
paternalism, 67, 68
patient-doctor relationship, xiii, 5, 8, 13, 67, 69, 73, 75, 78, 140. *See also* lay-professional interactions
patient knowledge, 63, 68, 69, 72, 73, 81, 94, 100, 134, 140
patient narrative, 45
patients: authoritative, 13; and compliance, 13; expert, 73

pellagra, 35
perinatal mortality, 52, 54
pharmaceutical industry: in development of consensus, 36, 107; in direct-to-consumer advertising, 71, 74, 85, 100; over-the-counter medications, 51, 71; in promotion of diagnoses, 10, 49, 94, 100, 109, 141. *See also specific corporations*
phrenology, 43
physiognomy, 43
PMS, 113
political diagnoses, 79–80
post-traumatic stress disorder, 11, 88–90, 94
premenstrual dysphoric disorder, 148
premenstrual syndrome, 113, 148
premenstrual tension, 113
prenatal diagnosis, 131
proanorexia, 95, 105
pro-choice movement, 51
Procter and Gamble, 107, 111
professional status, 6–10
pro-life movement, 51, 53
prostate cancer, 101, 129, 140
pseudodisease, 128
psychiatry: as arbiter of the unexplained, xiii, 30, 35, 83; need to assert professional status of, 7, 22, 23, 30, 32, 33; as political tool, 79–80
psychoanalysis, 34
psychosis, 95
psychosomatic disorders, 30, 85. *See also* medically unexplained symptoms
PTSD, 11, 88–90, 94

Read Codes, 29
resource allocation, xiii, 4, 5, 6, 7, 29, 37, 52, 67, 88, 98, 140–141
Rosenberg, Charles, 7, 30, 35, 45, 50, 60, 83, 139, 148

sarcoidosis, xii
scales, 44, 45
Schneider, Joseph, 8, 60, 67, 88, 97
screening, 126–131
self-depreciating personality disorder, 114
self-diagnosis, 8, 49, 51, 70–73, 94

Sexual Interest and Desire Inventory–Female, 107–108
sexuality: female, 9, 98, 101–104, 112–116; homosexuality, 3, 33; libido, xvi, 4
sickle cell anemia, 118
social constructionism, 40–41
social expectations, 5
social framing, of diagnoses, 2–4, 14, 39, 41, 59–61, 98
social movements. *See* health social movements
speculum sine macula, 47
Spitzer, Robert, 34, 89
spotless mirror, 47
Star, Susan, 4, 12, 26, 34, 35, 36, 145
statin drugs, 128
Statistical Manual for the Use of Institutions of the Insane, 31
stigmatization, xiii, 38, 50, 78, 105, 130, 131, 145
stillbirth, xv, 51, 52, 53, 55, 56. *See also* fetal death
surrogate markers, 127–128
surveillance medicine. *See* screening
symptoms, 63–64, 66, 81, 123–125
Systemized Nomenclature of Medicine, 29

taxonomy, 6, 16, 17, 19, 20, 31, 64, 81, 92
technology, xvi, 66, 81, 107–108; ultrasound, 134; x-rays, 117, 123, 126, 135, 140
technoscientization, 120
Tiresias, 102
Tokelauans, 135
Tongans, 37
transformative moment, xii, 1–2, 26, 62
tuberculosis, 26

understudied and under-resourced populations: Cook Islanders, 37, 50, 135; Niueans, 50; Tokelauans, 135; Tongans, 37
unwanted childlessness, 4, 9, 21

vaginal yeast infection, 70, 72
verité au malade, 2
Vertinsky, Patricia, 10, 85, 113
veterans, 89, 90, 129
virtue, 47, 48

Ward, Katie, 74, 92, 93, 95, 105, 142
wastebasket diagnosis, 30, 83
weight tables, 44, 45
Willis, Thomas, 6
witchcraft, 3
women's health, 85

Zavestoski, Stephen, 5, 11, 68, 79, 90, 91
Zerubavel, Eviatar, 15, 18, 19, 35, 143
Zola, Irving, 8–9, 97

About the Author

Annemarie Goldstein Jutel is the director of research at the Graduate School of Nursing, Midwifery and Health at Victoria University of Wellington (New Zealand). She initially trained as a nurse in Nantes, France, and subsequently pursued undergraduate and then doctoral studies in physical education at the University of Otago (NZ). She resides in Wellington and Otago, New Zealand.